# The Homœopathic Proving
## of
# SPECTRUM

## GILL DRANSFIELD

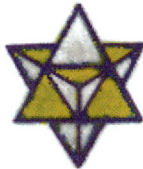

Penvith
Publishing

Published by
Penvith Publishing
Penvith Farmhouse
St. Martin – by – Looe
Cornwall
PL13 INZ

Email: gdransfield@penvithpublishing.co.uk
Web Site: www.gilldransfieldhomeopath.org.uk

ISBN  0 9538893-0-0


Printed by Launceston Printing Company
Dockacre Road, Launceston, Cornwall. PL15 8BN

Proof-read by Hilary Sawyer

Cover design by HIGGNOSIS and Gill Dransfield

Graphics on Theme Map by Graham Andrews

# A Moment of Focus

You are small yet powerful.
I know my sense of oneness overwhelms you.
I feel my life, my needs, my dreams,
You think yours –
And therein lies the difference.

We are both children of the Universe, You and I.
Our power when shared is multiplied.

I give you a gift,
The gift of light
And a calmness to keep it shining.

There is a gentleness in my strength.

A lightness of step and a lightness of thought –
Surrender to the lightness of body and spirit
And let your instinct be your guide.

Accept this gift and join with me,
Dance
And let the light be free.

Dee Laljee

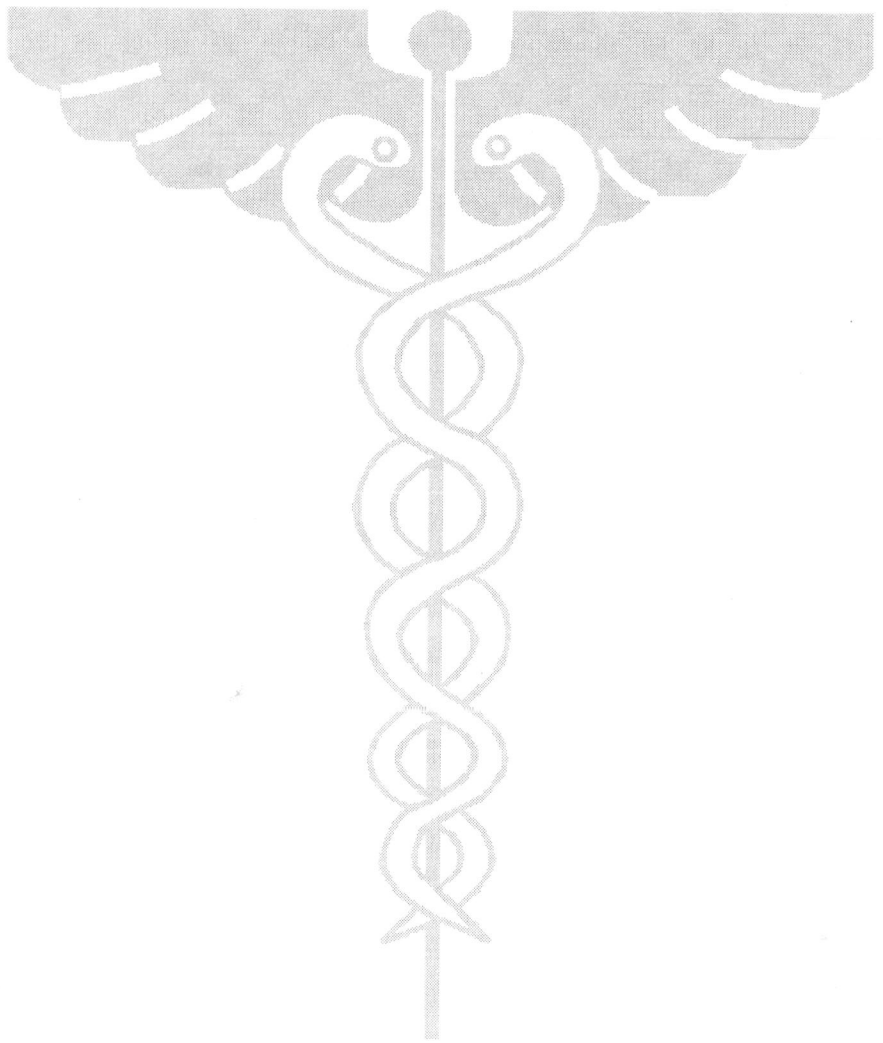

# Acknowledgements

Thank you, to John Morgan of Helios for your support.

Thank you, to Jeremy Sherr and his team at Dynamis; for giving us homœopaths who are foolish enough to embark on a proving, such a clear guide in the 'Methodology of Proving'

Thank you, to all the provers whose part in this I find particularly humbling considering all but two were non-homeopaths.

Thank you, to my son Kit for having the patience to teach me how to use the computer, so that I could write this thing up.

Thank you, to my son Luie, my little light bearer.

Thanks Robin for constant supply of tea, Gin {the rock} Skinner, Pat Neil {for leading us to the myth of Chiron} and last but by no means least Dee Laljee for bringing me back into focus just at that point when I was feeling totally overwhelmed.

To those that are close that form the framework.

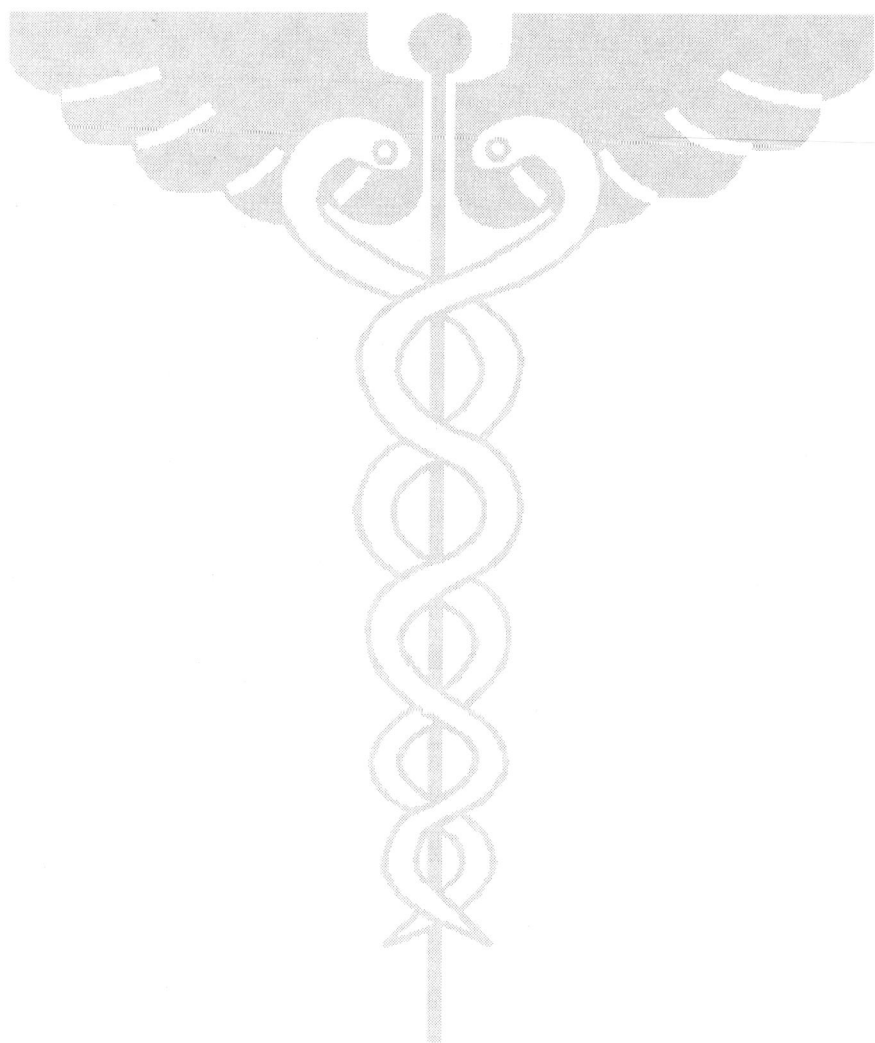

# Contents

# Introduction

**During** a visit to India in Spring '95 I had the idea to prove the colours of the visible spectrum. A highlight of this trip was to find myself in a stunningly beautiful Himalayan valley, where each day I visited the meditation garden of the Russian artist and philosopher Nicholas Roerich. Over the May Day celebrations I had a series of images whilst in a meditative state. In one I found myself walking in the valley accompanied by elves and faeries, not diminutive creatures but tall shimmering light beings. One of them gave me a wooden box, inside which were seven phials of colour, the seven colours of the visible spectrum. Also in the box were seeds and a handful of earth. (A symptom of a misspent youth with Tolkien, perhaps!) Over the next few months this became a recurrent image in dreams and meditation, so I decided to do something about it.

**After** much deliberation with both my father and Misha Norland, I finally contacted my old friend Katherine Boulderstone at Helios. Between us we agreed that what was needed were a prism, sunlight and bottles of medicating alcohol, which were exposed to the various colours. Spectrum itself was made up by Laura Russell, also of Helios, who used a transmitter quartz to shine a complete spectrum on a bottle of medicating alcohol. This was then made up into potentized remedies.

By March '96 we had started proving our first colour. All but two of the provers were non-homoeopaths, which was intentional, with a core of six provers who met regularly as a meditation group. The proving was conducted as a classical Hahnemannian proving. I did play around with different potencies in the first couple of provings but didn't notice any benefit and my experience is that 30c potency gave a full proving picture.

**One** of the daunting things about a proving is how complete the experience is, how inner and outer realities merge. Sometimes it becomes too much and we want to stop. Spectrum, like a number of recent provings - Plutonium for one - has been difficult to antidote. Coffee aggravated, and giving constitutional rx. seemed to take down the intensity, but it was still felt to be lurking in the background. Provers began to believe that they really were very ill; some believed this was terminal. This is the nature of the proving which has a picture of a very lowered vital force, an inability to throw off symptoms, indicative of a weakened immune system, a picture that is becoming more prevalent among today's population.

**Without light** there is no life. All higher life forms depend upon light. Plant life, which forms the basis of our food chain, photosynthesises light and stores it in the cells. Seventy per cent of the light we take into our bodies is through the eyes, where it is picked up by the light-sensitive pineal gland. Light informs the hypothalamus, autonomic nervous system and endocrine system and these three systems co-ordinate most of the homeostatic functions of the body. Does light inform the vital force?

Mankind has recognized since time began that sunlight is vital to our health and well being; yet modern man is now being warned to keep out of the sun. We work in offices with artificial lighting and are depriving ourselves of natural full spectrum light, and in the proving we can see the result.

**Light deprivation,** first noticed in night workers, can cause such symptoms as confusion, disorientation, irritability, loss of appetite, chronic tiredness and reduction of immune system.

We also recognize that the lack of sun in winter can cause a very debilitating depression in seasonal affective disorder (SADS), all symptoms found in this remedy.

When our immune system is compromised our boundaries thin and we become oversensitive to external impressions. There is a nervous, 'on edge' quality to this remedy coupled with a profound tiredness. It is not difficult to see how spectrum can be thought of in cases of ME or post-viral fatigue and I have successfully treated such cases with spectrum in my practise. I also recently had a case that presented with viral meningitis, and a history of chronic fatigue due to long term, unresolved crisis, which responded remarkably well to a dose of Spec. 30c. This patient wants to give her daughter Spec. as a prophylaxis against viral meningitis!

**I feel** it also relevant to mention that the idea for the proving coincided with one of the most difficult periods of my life. I had fallen into the abyss, the infamous 'long dark night of the soul' and was forced to look at some of my major 'issues'. Amidst all of this I fell prey to flu. Superficially this lasted three weeks but I didn't completely recover for another four years. It wasn't until I began to collate the provings that I realized how I had inadvertently prolonged my crisis, as the provers' symptoms were mirroring my own. The feeling is of being at a transition point. Many provers found themselves dealing with deeply ingrained blocks. Main issues arose relentlessly and had to be dealt with. With Spectrum we are not dealing with the energy of a substance but the pure energy prior to crystallization into form. This is a deeply miasmatic remedy.

**To understand** the deeper workings of a remedy we often turn to the myths and archetypes. The myth of Chiron has for us become synonymous with the proving and was discovered by one of the provers, an astrologer, when she decided to cast natal charts for each of the provings. Both the myth and the astrology can be found in the appendices.

It seems quite coincidental that within weeks of completion my father broke his thigh and I had to drop everything and go to his aid. It was a very worrying time but also a good lesson for my father, who came face to face with his mortality when a week after the fall he was rushed into hospital with an embolism in his chest. Happily, as a result of his experience he has a restored lust for life.

I deliberately kept away from any literature on colour and light during the proving in order to give myself a fair chance at experiencing the colours and not intellectualising. I felt it was important to do a double blind testing for the same reason. It's good to go into a proving without maps, it's a journey that unfolds.

**Once** we had finished proving I began to research the nature of light and many fascinating discussions were had on the biochemistry, physics, metaphysics…We went off into hyperspace – very symptomatic of this remedy! I began to write some of this up but soon realized that it deserved a book of it's own [this is a future project] and was not essential in understanding the basic nature of this remedy.[1] A proving is only the first draft and I feel that I have only scratched the surface. I am eagerly awaiting feed back from all you brilliant homoeopaths out there – please e-mail me.

When Misha commented wryly that this was my life's work I thought he was joking. I should have known better! I was trying to have all eight provings completed and out by now but being an eternal optimist I badly underestimated the time scale. So I've decided for now to publish Spectrum alone as it has shown, and will show, what a fundamental remedy it is.

Gill Dransfield DSH, RSHom.

[1] A brief synopsis of the science of light can be found in appendix 4.

# List of Provers

Prover No.1  — female — Spectrum 30c

Prover No.2  — female — Spectrum 30c

Prover No.3  — female — Placebo

Prover No.4  — female — Spectrum 30c

Prover No.5  — female — Spectrum 30c

Prover No.6  — male  — Placebo

Prover No.7  — female — Spectrum 30c

Prover No.8  — female — Spectrum 30c

Prover No.9  — female — Spectrum 30c

Prover No.10 — female — Spectrum 30c

Prover No.11 — female — Spectrum 30c

Prover No.12 — female — Spectrum 30c

Prover No.13 — female — Spectrum 30c

Prover No.14 — female — Spectrum 30c

Prover No.15 — female — Spectrum 30c

Prover No.16 — female — Spectrum 30c

Prover No.17 — female — Placebo

Prover No.18 — male  — Spectrum 30c

Provers took no more than six doses over two days, stopping the remedy as soon as symptoms appeared.

## Abbreviations

D = Day

M = Month

D- = Day before proving started i.e. D-5 = Five days before start of proving.

5

# SPECTRUM

## Mind and Emotions

Symptoms

Symptoms prior to proving

16. Felt very tuned into the animals today. I always talk to the cats and the dog, but somehow felt their communion with me. Noticed the animals, I was outside, the birds and the way they fly singly or in pairs. Noticed the feeling of connection. Busy day.  D-5

16. Feeling a bit lazy today. Walked dog without the usual gust and energy. Not tiredness so much as heaviness, as if conscious of body weight and the heaviness of physicality. Having to carry the body around when the spirit could float about without it.

Contented feeling as the day progressed. Ready for bed earlier than usual.  D-4

16. Very aware of all animals still, even a little fly or bug, even a worm crossing my path. It's as if I have a stronger recognition of these specks of life as somehow being as big and as important as my own is to me. The cats definitely seem to be talking to me. I feel tuned into their looks and noises, as if I can almost translate their looks and sounds literally.

More energy but still a dreaminess.  D-3

16. Went to see my dad in a holiday cottage. Spent sometime looking at the owner's owls, a sanctuary for squirrels, bird's, etc. I felt so connected to the owls. They seemed to be able to communicate with me and I with them, a real kinship. It felt quite unnerving. They seemed to literally be putting thoughts into my head and me sending them messages back. Very powerful.

Snowy owl said, "I'm scared, I don't like it. I don't know what to do." I tried to reply with calmness, then the aviary man said, "This owl is new here, it's been a bit skittish." Eagle owl said, " This is not the place for me really. I am bigger than you. I maybe in this cage but I have my pride." I said that I recognised his grandeur and majesty. I did not feel above it because it was in captivity. I also wanted to say that to be out in the wild at the moment would mean a short life.

The aviary man told us that this pair of Eagle owls, has been with him for sometime and although the female lays eggs, they never hatch, so they are infertile. It just fitted with what I heard him say about his pride!     D-2

16.     Driving home suddenly felt overwhelmed with grief, a real sadness. I could not stop the tears streaming down my face. I couldn't think where this was coming from or why. But I had to release it. A part of me somehow relishing this sadness [Bizarre.] Still felt sensitive all evening.     D-1

16.     Feeling slightly separate from people, again a strange feeling for me. I respond and act as I normally do but sense a sort of distance. Almost as if I'm standing a little outside my body and watching. Perhaps it is an awareness of spirit. A jay flew in front of me up the lane as if leading me. I could not grasp what it meant, but it felt like an omen, a good one. Something to do with precious moments and drops of wisdom and trust.

Have absolutely no interest in work [Traveller stuff.] This is not unusual, but today it felt as if it was sliding over me like water off a duck's back. I preferred to look out of the windows, noticed the colour of the sea in the distance. Really felt close to the trees and somehow befriended by them.

Still don't have masses of bubbly energy, odd for me. But I do feel relaxed and almost like nothing can harm me. Slightly cocooned or sitting in a bubble, watching the world outside but not somehow in what most people call reality. Much more in a spirit place.     D-1

## Proving symptoms

### First few minutes

14. Immediately on taking remedy experienced a rush of energy. The patterns on my wallpaper came out in 3D, they had texture. It was as if I was tripping.

1. On taking the remedy energy became visible. I could see energy in the room, radiating from the centre of the other provers' bodies and also mine. My head became very clear.

10. I am not aware of my body. It is as if I've become an onlooker.

5. My head felt spinney and I experienced the feeling of not participating. I was observing - uncommunicative.

### First half hour

Gen.
(7,8,17, Feel totally detached from everything.
5,1,14.)

10. Feeling of detachment from the group.

5. I'd love to go out and go for a hard walk.

10. My mind feels so clear, analytical. I could sit an exam right now.

8. Feel very warm from inside. Could also feel other's warmth. Warm panicky feeling from my heart centre, but no palpitations.

8. Feel totally balanced, quiet. All my aggression has gone.

Gen.
(7,8, Feel heavily relaxed, tired.   D1
17,5.)

17. I felt so energised I thought I could fly, as if in a heightened state of awareness, all charged up.   D1

9. Surging feeling from abdomen. Subtle but not weak, sense of 'shift': feel as if on a subtle level something has moved, giving way to greater balance.   D1

9.     Feel very fiery and energetic.   D1

16.    Feeling quite lethargic most of day but very insightful. When counselling    clients today I felt very clear and prepared to allow my intuitive side more strength. Seemed to <u>really</u> be aware of people in their lives and what their lives are like.   D1

1.     Could sit and give a lecture, as a superior teacher type.   D1

10.    I feel such disappointment in my marriage. I've been so let down.   D1

8.     Quite a physical day sorting and shifting stock, felt good physically.   D2

8.     I felt happy planning a nice meal to celebrate 'our' anniversary. But things went horribly wrong. We didn't argue, but a <u>long</u> discussion followed. I thought he was going to leave and felt incredibly miserable at the thought of never seeing him again. Emotionally I felt gutted. I could also feel his pain…

       …I felt hollow inside. My right shoulder neck area became painful again.   D2

12.    Feel a heightened clarity of 'vision'. All my senses feel acute, very sensitive.   D2

12.    Feel calmer and content within myself. Not bothered by what 'they' think. I'm going to get on with it, not care and do it anyway. Full of positive thoughts and of hope, once you trust it's all there.   D2

9.     I feel balanced, feeling of connection and energy is flowing. Optimistic.   D2

9.     Can see and trust, where things are going. Increased understanding. I feel organised as if I've enough time to do everything, without stress or rushing. I'm motivated but without 'hyperness'. Everything is falling into place: acceptance.   D2

16.    Calmness through the day, but a slight "out-of-bodyness" too.   D2

7.     Been very irritable, snapping at people.   D2

17. Feeling irritable, mumbling to myself all day. Grump-grump-grrrh-under the breath.   D2

10. I've been a bit irritable-niggley underneath. A bit terse with mother-in- law, I'm not suffering fools. Everyone is a fool!   D2

12. There is a lot of hostility and intimidation at work at the moment. A lot of stress, people not coping. A lot of people being ill.   D2

8. I've been waking up with butterflies in my stomach. Feeling very insecure of my finances.   D2

12. I couldn't face work - travelling to work. So I took the day off and I'm doing things at home, where it's nice and quiet.   D3

17. Have been aware of the presence of 'entities' around my bed at night. They are dark, shadowy, alien. I feel as if I'm being invaded. When I lie on my front I'm aware of the possibility of anal probing. It's as if I'm an abductee, being taken somewhere without my knowing. It's extremely frightening.   D3

17. I feel unhurried. I won't be hurried.   D3

8. Felt deeply depressed all day, moved lots of furniture around, felt better for it. But I feel a sense of impending doom. It could be anything, accident, money problems. Basically my future feels unsure. I feel a lot of fear.   D3

8. Whilst driving I felt very light headed, like I wasn't really here. Went to Tai chi, which is usually grounding, but still felt unbalanced.   D3

8. Nothing has rocked my emotional boat, as this, for ages. Later in evening experienced fluttering in chest/heart area.   D3

8. Who am I? What is my status? How far have I come? Where am I? Where am I going? What is expected of me? Am I worthy? What are my responsibilities? What is my position in a relationship? What kind of woman am I? What do I feel?

Am I looking after my emotional needs...and more?   D3

5.       Very busy day. Very energetic physically. Oozed confidence during a workshop and college lesson I was taking.   D3

8.       I feel like I'm at some kind of crossroads in my life.   D3

8.       Am I at some kind of crossroads in my life? I'm having water dreams -emotional insecurity. Crossroads, travelling fast down roads, getting lost. Some kind of crisis is happening or suggested.   D3

16.      Colours on the moor and down at the river really stunning, hitting the eyes almost in cleanness and brightness. A little bird, the dipper, came to say hello down at the river. Never seen one there before, it felt like an acknowledgement. It honoured me, I honoured it, no words. Still the feeling of being slightly out of body, more aware of the spirit, all day.   D3

1.       I have been very irritable, bitching in my head, not outwardly (unusual). I've been very shitty to people at work but not telling them. I've capped it.On returning home there was dog shit all over my house.   D3

17.      My partner is moody, irritable, argumentative and critical this morning and I've been avoiding him, as I don't want to fight. Instead I went for a walk and got soaked. My heart was bleeding and I wanted to cry. Why am I locked into such an unhappy situation, living with someone who is constantly dissatisfied. I became very down. My heart felt heavy. I arrived home to find that my red scarf had bled onto my favourite jumper, in the region of my heart!   D3

17.      Feel slightly irritable, critical towards friends and family. Very disappointed with my life.   D3

10,17.   Feel detached from others' moods / emotions or if slightly affected regain balance again very quickly and easily.   D3

9.       Excessive irritability. Back is bad too. Aching, painful, stiff.
         D3

16. Very late night so may have effected day. Very close to tears all day. Feeling ultra sensitive but ready to really sob and cry, as if the tears were waiting in the wings ready to flood in at the merest hint of a reason. (I was sent two lots of red roses in the last two days, from distant men that I rarely see and have no relationship with (sexual). Very strange, but very nice. Am I more open and vulnerable?   D3

10. My daughter and husband are finally talking, they are beginning to reconcile a feud of over two years. I'm feeling so much more positive and hopeful about the future.   D4

17. I've had a very busy productive day, but by evening my legs were aching. Finger joints stiff and swollen, also stitching pain in region of heart, radiating left.   D4

17. I want to be at home.   D4

17. I'm totally indecisive at the moment.   D4

8. Weather: sunny at first, rain later becoming heavy, just about describes my mood today. Getting more and more gloomy.   D4

8. Feel tired, overburdened. Sad about past and unsure about the future.   D4

12. At a workshop yesterday it was suggested that we should work honestly. I always do that and get into trouble. There is so much rivalry and competition. We are all equal or we are nothing.   D4

12. I feel there has been a fundamental shift after Diana's death. We can work together in the collective unconscious. Not doing it for personal gain. Following our intuition.   D4

12. I have noticed a lot of electromagnetic activity. There's an energetic thing going on. Things electrical are breaking and doing odd things.   D4

12. I feel calm, lack of fear. A sort of trust in life and dare I say survival. Whilst talking to a friend of possible tidal waves to come due to all the earth changes, I realised I am not that

bothered.  D4

9. Have a sense that this remedy works in stages, with a tidal wave effect. I can feel something building up.  D4

16. Less sparky energy again, not like me. Much more floaty, head feels heavy and noticing the body as opposed to the spirit. Everything seems less urgent, no panic, slightly distanced from me.  D4

16. The animal/bird connection is very strong but I am beginning to be more used to it all and the feelings have become less remarkable as they have been with me for so many days now. The dog, the cats and I have real conversations, they are now wordless and it is more like a knowing and a passing, difficult to put into words because it is communication without words. Even on a practical level the dog gets up, I know he's thirsty but the water needs changing. The cat comes down the stairs, I know he has come to see where I am, not to go out or to eat. It feels very normal and I've almost stopped registering it as different.  D4

1. I feel very creative.  D4

5. Felt livid with my mother for not helping me when I was so sick. She just changed the subject and I couldn't get the anger out of me.  D4

1. Feeling antagonism towards my daughter. Petty stuff really getting to me. Injustice towards me, felt I'd been dealt a poor hand. But I had to keep my mouth shut until I could find the right time to talk about it. Felt I had to suppress my anger. So I went to the moors, I needed the space to get away from it all. D4

17. Want to get on and do things, but just can't get going. Becoming adept at displacement activity.  D5

8. Feel great fear, like impending doom. Any moment my security could be ripped from me. Like a rug going to be pulled from under.  D5

8.     Having lots of feelings about the past. I also feel there is a new path for me but I'm not conscious if it. But I know there's a change coming and I feel more fear than excitement. A BIG change. I've been looking back on my life with feelings of regret.   D5

17.    I've been reviewing my life. Really trying to work out who I am, what I want to do with my life, where I want to be.   D5

8.     I've rearranged my house. Clearing up, sorting out both at work and at home.   D5

16.    I feel in touch, connected and quite high spiritually. It is strange for me to feel this lack of spark. It has subdued some of my practical creative energy. I'm much too floaty to get into that. Just loving the relaxedness of it all but a bit like "being ill" for me in some ways physically, because I'm so used to the Aries impulsiveness, the bursts of energy. The remedy has shone light upon another facet of me, but not just me, of life.   D5

8.     Confused day, disorganised. I 'felt' disorganised but actually accomplished quite a bit. Cleared a cupboard and cleared out the house.   D5

10.    I've had a busy, industrious and satisfying day.   D6

8.     I'm waking up in a grumpy mood.   D6

17.    Finding it difficult to concentrate.   D6

8.     Don't want to go to work. Feel horrible, grumpy and out of sorts. I felt so non-specific miserable.   D6

8.     Feel as if I'm undergoing some crisis but I have no idea what it is. I feel I need to get to grips with my strange dreams and huge fears.   D6

5.     Feeling very vague about things, a feeling of can't be bothered. My head feels spinney when I grab some college work or a book, a feeling of brain overload.   D6

8.     Have a strong feeling that I'm coming into money or "treasure".   D7

17,7,10. I'm standing up for myself, not in a nasty way. Becoming more assertive.   D7

4.   I've had a very physical week. Riding three times. Once on a very dangerous and out of control feeling horse. Nearly had an accident, almost fell on top of a car. Was very frightened. Monday night went singing and did a dance class. Felt good about being so physical.   D7

13.   Have broken up with boyfriend of five years. Now feeling very sad, lonely, all alone. Nothing to look forward to.   D7

17.   Feeling lucky, as if I'm going to win some money.   D8

17.   I'm finding work very tiring. Need a lot of rest.   D8

8.   Felt irritable on arrival at work. Everything is a mess, so untidy. I'm irritable because it isn't the way I like it. Control again.   D9

8.   Experienced surges of warmth/heat again throughout the day. Ideas for interesting things, creative things bubbling up inside me.   D9

13.   My son (15) has visited his father for the first time since his father walked out on us when my son was nine. The beginning of peace talks between them!   D10

7.   I've been pulled to gold (unusual) and I've been wearing a gold jumper all week.   D10

8.   I feel out of sorts (have had three late nights in a row). Have been noticing exhaust fumes lately. Aware of breathing them in. Chest felt tight, I felt poisoned by them, like they were infiltrating my body, down my tubes into my lungs, spreading out across my chest. I wanted to breathe fresh clean air. Later I was plagued by nausea and it hurt when I breathed out.   D11

1.   I'm in bed with flu, so I've decided to talk to my nephew who is in prison. I record myself telling him how I came to my spiritual path. When I had finished I felt well again and next week I'm going to Prague.   D11

1.     I've been noticing big cats - panthers, both in meditation and outer reality.

   There is a new lion at Newquay zoo and the beast of Bodmin has been sighted again. Is it a Black Panther?  D11

17.     I've been attracted to gold (normally a silver person). Bought a gold jumper from the Oxfam shop and have worn it all week. D11

7.     Attracted to bright blue and electric cobalt blue. Whilst driving home last night, cats eyes seemed more gold than silver with connecting lines of blue-electric cobalt blue.  D11

5.     I can live alone. I can cope. I am independent, strong, self - sufficient. I don't need him (husband). I've changed.  D12

1.     I am fighting back 'him indoors'. Standing up for myself. I've never done this before.  D12

17.     Feeling confident about the state of the world. Things will turn around. Things will change, are changing for the better. More and more people are waking up to the truth and are doing something to change things.  D12

17.     Feelings of impending disaster, but with it a lack of fear, an inner calm and total trust in a power, greater than me.  D13

17.     Since taking the remedy there seems to be more hope around. D14

17.     I'm so tired I cannot think. It's all too much of an effort. My thinking is confused. I lack any clarity. I feel overwhelmed by others even the sound of their voices can become a pressure. I want to be alone to find peace, silence and tranquillity.  D14

10.     Work, work, work yet feeling fine, in control and able to cope with anything. Not feeling tired.  D14

12.     My motivation is to do the things I enjoy doing.  D14

12.     Communication has become very powerful. The general public can now access ALL the information. Case of Louise Woodward - the people were not having an injustice and got

together and did something about it. Once people know the truth, they won't allow the lie to be. D14

8,4,7. Non-specific down feeling. D14

17. Feeling down and irritable. Feeling dissatisfied, old grievances coming up and OUT. D14

10. Feeling optimistic, things are on the way up. Good positive feelings in general. D14

12. Feeling very optimistic at the moment. Feel like I've turned a corner. D14

17. I feel very vulnerable - psychically drained/depleted. It's as if my energy body is not there or has become very thin. There is too much going on around me -noise, radio, T.V., people talking at me - telephone constantly ringing. It's all too much. I've become hypersensitive to external stimulus. I want to escape. D15

17. I am wanting/needing time on my own. Time for ME. Time to rest my body, giving me time to think my thoughts. Other people are draining my energy. D15

10. Feel psychically drained, as if my energy body is not there. D15

17. Last night in bed I felt as if I was falling in to unconsciousness and death. I saw a long tunnel of white light and decided to let go and fell into the tunnel. It felt good, natural and so familiar. D15

4. Have managed to remain suprisingly cheerful so far, but this was too much. I cried and felt better. D15

10. This remedy seems to be a synthesis of all the other seven remedies we have done. D16

4. Found myself during relaxation on a beautiful Greek island looking at the sea, smelling herbs. I felt very powerful in this place.

My mother in-law phoned to say her sister had died this

morning. Upset, she had gone for a walk on the beach and seen a rainbow. This made her feel comforted. After discussing the significance of rainbows with her, she said to me "I knew you'd understand about the rainbow." D16

4.  Stayed awake late (unusual) reading Louise Hay and deciding to change my life. D16


4.  Woke feeling much better, walked dogs, swept, tidied up and went shopping. Too much. Was so tired I fell asleep on the sofa in the afternoon.[v. sweaty(smelly), pain in rt. hip and rt. groin]

Regret overdoing things.[sore, dry throat, catarrh and discomfort in upper chest.] Uncomfortable flashback to exactly 2 years ago, the time of my horrible illness-M.E. I'm trying to make this circle feel like an undoing. Have been quite successful so far. Was even able to get out the dreaded rag rug into which I worked so much fear and sickness back then. The hope was that I could finish it this time and get rid of my sickness forever. It feels as though, while it still lurks unfinished in my cupboard, it could jump out and get me. D17

## Each November.

November brings the sharp-edged fear of death.
I see it lurking in the earliest
Christmas decorations, hear it's rasp on
TV sherry ads., catch it skulking in
corners  giving off an odour something
between sulphur and pine. From fireworks night
to choosing the tree I drowned screaming in
midwinter slime. Now when the light is low
and the crow caws and the world hunkers down,
the cold grey echoes and the taint of air
turn my lungs to jelly. I die again.
Looking at my last Christmas, I was sure.

I made each card with care from silk and glass
on ripped art paper with a jagged edge
and lay awake at night, lungs full of tears,
writing of mermaids. And when Christmas came
Death did not. Not that time. I breathed again.
Each Winter as the earth turns and the lights
go down sooner I know that I can mark
Christmas in red the same day every year.
But as for Death, it's advent is less clear.

8.     Feeling tired, drained of energy last few days. Less to do with late nights and more to do with lack of 'own time'. I feel depleted and everyone seems to be drawing energy out of me. I feel impatient and resentful. Other drivers annoy me. Some people are getting under my skin. I long to be on my own for a couple of days.    D17

8.     I feel the need to be outside in Nature, by myself to replenish my energy levels. A picture grew in my mind of towns and cities filled with people feeding off each others' energy and getting all jangled and confused. How healthy to live in the countryside.    D17

8.     My grandson (2) talked of rainbows, moons and stars constantly today.    D17

8.     Webs and nets are coming up for me lately. I have to make some, draw some… I feel as if I'm caught in a web, a net, a trap at present. Why don't I consciously weave a web for myself, a web of destiny?    D17

18.    Brilliant meditation which clarified some of my recent problems. My irritation with others is caused by control issues. I get annoyed when I can't control some situations and so experience irritation.[My Saturn transit is causing me to focus on this. Saturn likes structure, discipline and responsibility but can be too controlling, restrictive.] I'm trying to control minor, petty, unimportant areas of my life, but have no control over myself.

I allow myself to become depleted of energy- go to bed too late, agree to do so much for others and pretend to be easy going about it .Yet, I know it wears me out. Why don't I take proper care of myself? Take control of myself. Be responsible for myself.   D18

8.     Went to bed last night feeling dreadful. I'm not really physically tired or even mentally tired; I feel psychically drained. I felt this way three years ago when a friend stayed. She questioned me constantly and every time I answered she disagreed with me and criticised what I did. I felt her to be so judgmental that I stopped answering and began withdrawing into myself. I realised afterwards that she'd been stealing my energy.

Went to an exhibition yesterday and I think it compounded my feelings, too many people, too much going on.   D20

8.     Felt better today, although still pretty impatient/intolerant towards others.   D21

17.    Maniacally busy at the moment. My body is not keeping up with my mind.   D22

12.    I'm very, very busy. I'm on top of a wave.   D24

12.    It's been such a grey day, I'm so aware of the lack of light.   D24

Gen.
[4,8,17,    Feel as if my energetic body / energy level is depleted, has as
12,7,10.]   become thin.   D24

8.     I need space to think, to go off and digest things.   D25

Gen.
[5,7,8,17,4.] Becoming a hypochondriac.   D25

8.     I don't want to argue with my boyfriend. It is a waste of time, and it drains you.   D25

8.     Sick of constant rain, day after day. Two days ago we suffered thunder and lightning for hours and persistent rain, which caused freak flooding. I long to lie in the sun and soak up some good energy.   D25

13.    Feel like I'm going to collapse, due to dizzy spells. With this, a fear of heart problems - heart block - angina. I'm terrified of dying. I feel I might have an incurable disease.    D27

13.    Been feeling absolutely worn out. My limbs feel like lead. Wake up at night thinking I'm going to die.    D27

8.    For the last few evenings I have found projects to do rather than watching T.V, as I'm convinced it sucks energy out of me.    D27

13.    Keep hoping that the next man I meet will be the one, my soul mate.    D27

17.    Feel as if I'm in a different dimension. Having feelings / sensations even images that are impossible to describe / rationalise. It's as if the veil between reality and dream has thinned and I can voyage out into infinity.    M1

17.    Feeling of uncertainty in an unfamiliar territory. As if newly born, slowly, shakily focusing in on a new world. Like a butterfly fresh out of a cocoon, slowly unfurling my wings. M1

17.    After an ultrasound examination, felt a tangible change in myself and later felt very tired and invaded. The area that had been observed ached.    M1

9.    I keep seeing/hearing birds, lots of birds. I'm sure they are always there, but I'm now aware of them, wren, buzzard, snipe, jay and owls.    M1

18.    Terrified of losing my wife, being let down again as I was by my first wife.    M1

14.    Feeling grouchy, a definite anger thing just under the surface. M1

1.    Have felt the presence of dark forces/entities around me at night in bed. They do not feel good and make me feel great fear. I have to make a huge effort to dispel them.    M2

17.    Feel as if I'm in a dream. Lack of concentration, slow

comprehension due to being 'somewhere else'.
Mentally away with the faeries, yet getting on and doing on a practical level.   M2

8,17.   Felt as the action of the remedy began to recede I began to ground.   M2

17.   Feeling old. Feel as if I'm looking old. My hands look old. M2

17.   Mentally alert. Organised to the extreme. Generally life running smooth and I don't feel pressurised, which is unusual so close to Christmas!   M2

17.   Feeling really dragged down, tired and washed out. Overwhelmed by constant pain and constant tiredness. Felt so tired today I had to stay in bed almost all day.   M2

17.   Felt as if I was connected to the stars and one day I would return home.   M2

4.   Felt a sense of foreboding after the hurricane winds hit England. M2

5,8,1,17.   Excited by the storms. Compelled to go out and step into them. M2

1.   I was pulled first to the moor and then to the sea, where there were waves of 100 ft.   M2

17.   Driving out in the storm, avoiding falling branches, feeling excited, invigorated. Later walking along the coastal path watching in awe the mountainous waves and the boiling sea below.   M2

Gen.   Comment after the hurricane: - Felt humbled by the immense
[ 5,8,1,   strength of nature and how insignificant we really are. Feelings
17,12.]   of humility but above all a great reverence for Mother Earth. M2

17.   Feeling hot inside. My 'head is on fire', I feel really inspired, in a very creative mood.   M2

17.   Woke up thinking the world was on fire. All the forest fires

that are raging at the moment - Indonesia, Brazil, Australia - were joining up and consuming the world.  M2

4.      Got through Christmas trying to convince myself I was in love with my husband again. It worked for a while and we were quite happy.  M2

17.     Feel guilty when I take time off to rest/recover, a) Feeling like I'm skiving or b) Feeling pathetic, weak and unable to cope.  M2

8.      My head felt heavy and drowsy and I longed for fresh air, but it was pouring with rain and I couldn't have managed a walk with my painful legs.  M2

8.      I long for my own space, there are so many things I want to get stuck into and physically I want the bed to myself.  M2

8.      Felt frustrated, at times panicky, what was wrong with my leg?  M2

8.      I slept fitfully, strange images filled my head. It was as if my mind was a small room and images, thoughts, tastes, smells, sounds, things people had said, faces flew in and bounced off the walls and ceiling. They came in fast and furious. My head felt as if it would explode! A furnace burned inside me. I was sure if I opened my mouth, an onlooker would see it raging.

I guess I've been hallucinating as I kept seeing figures standing there, in the corner of my eye and when I turned they disappeared. I'd also seen bright sparks of light and fleeting, whirling patterns.  M2

8.      Feel like I need exercise.  M2

11.     I've been working very hard for weeks.  M2

11.     Constant thought/worry of being pregnant. I can't get it out of my mind. Like Chinese water torture, the thought constantly dripping.  M2

11.     Fear of ectopic pregnancy and huge fear of dying, having told no one I might be pregnant.  M2

11. Have been wanting to reduce my intake of alcohol, as I've been worrying recently that I may be addicted.  M2

17. Worrying that I may have become addicted, especially to smoking. So, making a conscious effort to clear my body of such toxins, in the hope of regaining some kind of energy level.  M2

7. I've been very busy lately.  M2

7. I'm feeling really glum at the moment and I'm on. I feel I'm letting myself down. Full of self-doubt and despair about my life. Before my period I was too depressed to do anything. Although there is a little bit in me saying this is an excuse for not getting on with what I've got to do. Feeling of being under pressure. I'm pathetic, a waste of time.  M2

7. Been feeling cloudy. I'm aware, but not quite sure what of.  M2

7. Finding that I'm being reminded to trust my instincts. Not taking notice and wishing I had.  M2

7. I set the curtains on fire in my front room. It was a windy night and I had candles burning too close to the curtains.  M2

17. Keep thinking the house is on fire. My son nearly set his room alight last night when a lit candle fell over onto his carpet. Luckily I had an impulse to check his bedroom and found it had burned a small hole in his carpet and was still aglow.  M2

7. Feeling very depressed and lonely. Feel I'm all alone, but haven't felt like going out. Just wanting to stay at home.  M2

7. My energy is sluggish. I feel heavy, dragging myself around. Can't be bothered to do anything.  M2

7. I feel bad as I am having awful feelings about my ex-boyfriend's new girlfriend. I feel like there is poison running around my body that won't come out. Have given up smoking, which has given me more energy.  M2

12. Feel livelier about things. No good just theorising, got to actualise. Work is fun and I've had a couple of good job offers. I like the students; even B. course leader flung his arms around me today. M2

12. I and everyone I know are feeling highly pressurised. There are not enough hours in a day and the days feel shorter. Weeks are whizzing past. M2

12. I went to see a psychic who said, "You're allergic to something. I can feel you, itchy". M2

12. My friend has terminal cancer. Helping her face her death has helped me face mine. M2

2. I feel much more in myself, much more vibrant.


8. I've been aware of what seems/feels like dark forces around me at night. It's very frightening. M2

8. I've been very dreamy, not really here. M2

14. I've been having suicidal thoughts. This is all too much, I want out. I seemed to lighten up, recover and then it happened again. The freedom of being free of the physical body. No self-pity, hatred or blame. M2

14. I feel as if this is a sort of transition of some description. M2

14. Looking back on these provings, if I were to do them again, I would do it differently, more scientific. But during the proving I was not in the headspace to be scientific. M2

17. Felt angry thinking of the abuse of power, individual and corporate. In particular the abuse of trust and the keeping of fundamental truths hidden from humanity. M2

17. Outbursts of anger, shouting and screaming uncontrollably at my husband. It felt as if this anger had been stored up for years and I felt better after, not sure about my partner. M2

17. I have spent the last few days crying. I feel so deeply hurt, all alone and loveless. M2

12.     I am compelled to read Col. Churchward's book, 'Sacred Teachings', inspired by books of the Golden Age. All about our origins. I want to know more and more.   M2

13.     Woke up in the night thinking that I'm going to die.   M2

Gen.
[2,7,8,4,17.] Feel as if my condition is incurable. Feel as if I'm dying.   M3

17.     Feel like I'm dealing with something on a deeply imprinted level{ past life / genetic inheritance stuff. }   M3

17.     Everything seems unreal.   M3

8.      I've been questioning myself deeply. What am I doing with my life? Questions of status / identity. Looking over missed opportunities. I'm not getting any younger.   M3

4.      The theme of the last few weeks has been ageing. My face, my body, my weight, my wrinkles. Fear of age. Fear that I will never have another lover. Fear that I look old and ugly. Fear that I will never have a proper career and that it is too late to start again. Fear that I have missed living. Fear of behaving and sounding middle aged. Fear of having been a nobody. Feeling ridiculous for not having a job, saying I'm an actor and not having acted for a long time. I was turned down at an audition for being too old last month. Fear that I will never be properly fit again. Fear that I will be too tired. I feel as though my life was full of grand possibilities that I missed through no fault of my own. I am unable or unwilling to accept responsibility for my own ignorance about how to live properly.
M3

4.      The thing is I've been waiting for forty years.
It'll happen soon. By the law of averages it must.
On occasions it has come right around the corner.
Sometimes when I've been looking for it
and others not, but I've heard it draw up
right outside. And go next door. Or to another room.

I've always kept a space for it.
I hurried my children through to make room.
There's plenty now, stacked with dusty pictures
for the time being, but I could breeze through
quick as anything and freshen things up.
I always keep an ear out for the telephone.

The thing is , and this is awful, but what if
it should have come while I was out ?
Or not looking ? Didn't recognise it ?
Or if it's invisible ? Here all the time,
waving at me just welling up
with all the waiting ? But that's too silly
to be true.    M3

17.    I'm feeling an increased nervous energy, coupled with great clarity of thought, great efficiency , drive and motivation. Truly getting things done. With it comes a slight apprehension that this is a high that will end in a fall. M3

10.    I'm having great clarity of thought.    M3

17.    Very excited about beginning a new challenge at work. Finding it difficult to switch off my brain. Feel hot constantly / nervous energy. Working until 3 am.    M3

17.    Mind busy with an endless stream of thoughts. My mind won't stop, it's particularly bad at night in bed, keeping me awake. M3

17.    There is too much on my mind. My mind will never stop. I've too much to do, I can't cope.    M3

17.    Nervous excitement, as if nervous system were turned up 300%.    M3

17.    Interminable restlessness night and day, can get no peace. Nervous exhaustion but can find no rest. I feel wired as if on speed, overexcited. I feel as if I'm burning up, it's as if my nerves are on fire. Heading for BURN OUT.    M3

1.    I haven't painted for thirty years, but I've enrolled in an Art's

class and there's no stopping me. I've got over a massive block.{curative} I'm also reading a very heavy book on the fallen angels. I've always had a huge block over reading. I'm trying to find the truth about our origins.   M3

8.  I've been feeling all charged up- electric.   M3

10. Racing feeling, like being on speed.   M3

17. Thrilled to be alive with all these possibilities with which to create. Projects, which have been blocked for two years, are finally happening. Enjoying making things, papier-mâché, and sewing. Feeling really inspired. Whilst modelling two angels for a piece I'm working on of the angel of night and the angel of day, I began to understand the concept of modelling from the clay. Ideas coming in to form.   M3

4.  Maniacally busy setting up the actors' co-op. Very worried about being able to cope with all the things I find I suddenly have to do. Feels like a potentially dangerous situation. I fear I will become ill.   M3

4.  I feel very tired at present; enthusiasm keeps me going in the office. Glad to have a life again. Feeling very positive.   M3

12. Feel a change in the air. I must take action. I need a new career direction, to earn my money in a different way, doing my own thing.   M3

7.  It keeps coming back. Shall I or not have another child. I think I'm pregnant and I really do want a child. They validate me. It's such a worthwhile thing to do.   M3

17. Feel a heightened ability to communicate and with it has come a feeling of validation.   M3

5.  I've been predominately full on, and then I get very tired feeling, extremes of energy, all or nothing.   M3

17. Began to feel as if I was finally getting better, then down again {Extreme exhaustion, agg. exertion, physical and mental. Feverish, sweaty, smelly sweat under arms and on feet. Sensitivity around waist, worse for clothes, pressure, heat, hot

head and forehead. Feeling as if I'm burning up.} M3

10. My memory has become extremely poor, both short and long term. I can't seem to hold any information. I love to read but there seems no point, as I'm remembering nothing of what I have just read. Forgetting how to spell and have poor memory for words in conversation. M3

7. My brain is just not working. M3

17. I've been totally indecisive for weeks, but it's getting so bad that I'm even breaking out in a cold sweat/palpitations, even trying to decide basics like what to wear in the morning and what to have for dinner tonight. M3

17. Huge desire for a month off, on a beach in the sun. A nice Greek island. M3

Gen. Huge desire for a holiday. M3

[1,7,4,10]

1. I've been pushing away me 'old man', just getting on with what I want to do, especially painting. M3

17,4. Since beginning this proving I have felt awkward around men. M3

8. I think the proving is finished and then I get more symptoms. M3

7. I feel debilitated, very worn down, really, really tired. It is almost impossible to keep awake all day. I have to lie down. M3

7. I feel emotionally open. M3

17. I'm beginning to worry that my brain isn't working properly. My thoughts are confused, my memory is abysmal, both short and long-term. My word recall is poor and I'm finding it impossible to organise my thoughts. It's as if someone has erased my memory banks. Is there something structurally or physiologically wrong, brain damage? As if a wire has been cut, a facility I had no longer there. I'm wondering whether people think I'm a bit slow. M3

7.     Feel like I'm becoming a cripple, always ill, and here I am training to be a therapist/healer. What use am I going to be to anyone?  M3

17.     Woke up this morning very depressed, despondent. I'm beginning to feel

gt. despair over my constant ill health. I cannot live with this, it's so limiting. I will never be well again. How can I help others when I'm always so poorly myself? Useless specimen. With it comes recurrent thoughts of suicide, wanting to drive my car at speed into a petrol / gas tanker.  M3

17.     Can't bear the thought of becoming a burden on anyone. I've always been so independent, I'm the one who usually does the caring.  M3

17.     Lately I feel exhausted when I'm in the company of others. It feels as if they are talking at me, very loud and I become very irritable. I vant to be alone with MY thoughts, my books. After visitors I have to go and lie down, they drain me.  M3

4.     Hard to be positive either about work or relationship, both are plumbing the depths at present. On Sunday morning, before I had even sat down to breakfast, I was in tears. On the surface it was a row over money, but I think it was something deeper, don't understand what yet. Felt as if I had been hit by some kind of emotional hammer and I'm still reeling two days later. M3

17.     I thought my appendix was going to burst due to the pain and heat in that region and I got very frightened. I thought about taking Belladonna, but was frightened it would make it happen. M3

17.     I thought my spleen was going to burst and I feared I might die.  M3

7.     I've been feeling emotionally open.  M3

10.     Now is a time I know I justifiably could feel angry, but I don't. Maybe it's coming out in my inflamed and infected arm, being

expressed only physically. M3

17. Become irritable and angry when my gall bladder / liver region hurts. M3

17. Overpowering sense of futility. What is the point of life? I'm normally very motivated, but at the moment can find no inspiration. Every idea I have I pick to pieces. It's all so flawed, I can find no worth in anything. Everything is doomed to fail, sheer hopelessness. Nihilism is becoming clear to me now. The feeling is of "eternal emptiness" that with which Mephistopheles threatens Faust. Even death is no way out. No one in this world can help me. M3

2. I'm feeling v. fearful, scared of being ill. Feel I've got something dreadfully wrong. I'm flipping in and out of reality. At times I think I'm losing it.

I feel like I've put something bad into my body. It's as if I'm recovering from a bad overdose. My solar plexus is way out - normally very strong. M3

7. Since taking this remedy I've begun a new relationship and I've been ill ever since.Because he's paying me attention. M3

4. I feel so let down by my marriage, so disappointed. But I've idealised love, I'm searching for the unobtainable, my other half, never wanting to give up hope. M3

17. Because of the hurt I feel towards my partner, I've been reviewing our marriage. I feel that I've been let down so many times, such deep disappointment. M3

7. I can't get away from this feeling of disappointment and hurt over my ex. He's really let me down, he's found a new girl friend and I'm gutted. M3

17. I've become obsessed with the idea of finding my twin soul. Someone I truly commune with. The idea is intoxicating, an unobtainable dream, but I can't let it go. M3

17,7. Wanting to wear purples and reds. M3

17.     Woke up and felt good, all my pains had gone. But as soon as my mind kicked in and I began to think of all the things I had to do and the pressure I felt I was under, the pains started. An aching tension in my heart and under rt. rib cage. It was as if someone had flicked a switch.   M3

8.     My brain hurts. I feel dehydrated, as if my brain is shrinking, drawing away from inside my skull. Is this what alcoholics feel like? My eyes feel as if they are sinking into the back of my skull.   M4

17.     I have been so oversensitive for the last three weeks. I feel as if I've lost a couple layers of skin.   M4

7.     My brain has gone at the moment.   M4

8.     My memory is bad. I'm forgetting words mid conversation. I can't remember how to spell simple words. I've been worrying that my brain isn't working properly.   M4

4.     My memory is non-existent at the moment.   M4

17.     Constant feeling of distance from everyone, family, friends, patients and reality. Sometimes with it a feeling of alienation, is there no one on my wavelength?   M4

4.     It's vague, nothing I can put my fingers on. Not physical, more a state of mind. Months ago I thought I'd got to grips with my life. Now my mind is like mud. I don't know. I can't think. I'm spaced out, in a different dimension. Feeling I might be going off somewhere.

    Thought I had control of it two weeks ago, thought I could pull myself back, but no. Total vague out.   M4

4.     I'm finding it impossible to write / think. I'm totally numb by the end of the day. Like a zombie, completely off my head. M4

4     I have to sleep.   M4

17.     Whilst walking the coastal path today, the world felt small under my feet.   M4

17.  I've distanced myself from my partner. I've no desire to be close to him. I run away into my room, surround myself with work or hide in yet another book.  M4

13.  I'm pushing people away, not people I'm close to, shedding superfluous people.  M4

17.  I've been reading obsessively, wanting to know everything. I know I should take more exercise but I'd rather read another book. Mentioned often how I wish I could unscrew my head and leave it with a book, while my body went out to play.  M4

10.  I'm reading and reading at the moment. I've got books on the go all around the house. I can't get enough information.  M4

13.  I feel as if my body is dragging down. I thought it was because there was too much happening in my life. It feels like this has been forever. My face and chest feel pulled down.  M4

4.  Still madly busy. Beginning to feel a real fear about my thirst for sleep. When I have to sleep, I have to sleep. Real exhaustion. This alternates with periods of frantic activity.  M4

4.  I'm having lucid, active periods. Interspersed with days when I am unable to stay awake, especially after physical activity. M4

17.  I've been looking towards death, in order to be transformed / reborn. I want a new life. I want to start again, fresh and healthy. M4

17.  I have been aware of the presence of angels, especially at night as I go to sleep, also while I'm meditating. They bring with them a feeling of total peace, calmness where all my fears dissolve. I feel protected by their love, divine love. When I'm walking in the countryside I feel their presence. I'm also aware of elementals, fairies, elves... I even feel like an elf myself sometimes, playing amongst the trees and flowers. Sometimes I see little flashes of light, from the corner of my eye or while I'm talking to someone, a flash of light over their head or in another part of the room. I feel a communication with another

realm almost all the time and that these 'entities' are in sympathy with me, working with me. But, with this comes a feeling of alienation. This is not the accepted, the norm. M4

17.    Feeling uncomfortable in my body. M4

17.    Memory is poor. I'm using wrong words (Mrs. Malaprop), and recall is slow. Confusing left from right Also get words and numbers around the wrong way, e.g. will copy a phone number from my ansaphone 847 when it should be 748. M4

17.    Forgetting words mid-sentence. Feel as if I've got holes in my memory, bits wiped off the tape. A virus in my brain. M4

17.    Feel unable to communicate all these thoughts. M4

17.    Feel thin, fragile, unnourished by my food. M4

12.    Something is not quite right; I feel we are close to the end of the world. We are definitely on the edge of something. M4

4.     My head is full of lead. I can't think straight, can't talk straight. Head is buzzing but feels dead. M4

4.     After riding, back at stables, inside dark and quiet. I met a man, ordinary man, felt drawn to him. It was like balm speaking to him, very quietly spoken, very calm. For a brief moment I felt recognition, a line connecting me to that inner calm. M4

8.     I'm experiencing mad hyper-energy, which is as physical as it is mental. With it comes a heat. Lots of ideas pouring in, can't sleep with it. I feel all charged up. M4

8.     I'm finding it difficult to communicate. I can't get through to anyone on the phone. No one in when I ring. I'm not being clear when communicating an idea or thought. M4

7.     There is a self-destruct thing going on for me. Last week, poisoned myself with whisky, drank much too much. M4

7.     Crying, bursting into tears. It all seems so hopeless. Feeling sorry for myself. Easily burst into tears, someone has just got to look at me. Everyone is getting on my nerves. I'm so tired. M4

12. Boundless energy. I come home from work, get something done and look for more. I'm very positive, very sociable at the moment. Enjoying life and feeling good. M4

1. Feeling better than I've done for many years. Dieting, walking, painting. Bought myself some new clothes and I feel good. M4

17. Giving up smoking, cutting out stimulants, eating wholesome food and exercising. Wanting to be clear in mind and body. Desire to be in peak health. M4

12. Life is speeding up; it's most unnatural. I haven't been cold all winter. It's been so unnaturally warm. M4

12. Crying in the car on my way home, from the bottom of my pit (day of solar eclipse). I felt suicidal. The pointlessness of existence. Doomed to do this forever and a day. No wonder I'm in tears of despair, I'm working at something that is not allowing my true creativity. We deny parts of ourselves and become paralysed.

The feeling is coming from the gut. It's like having a plug pulled out of my centre every time I go to work. M4

12. Knowing that I have got to trust my gut feeling and go for what allows my creative talents. Jumping into the unknown with only trust. M4

7. I'm so constantly tired I wonder if there is something seriously wrong with me. M4

17. Looking back over last months, since taking the proving, I have felt constant tiredness, extreme tiredness. Which leads to despondency and the feeling that I'll never be able to manage anything again. I'll always be like this. M4

4. I've been very awkward around men recently. M4

17. I can't find any clarity, floating in a sea of thoughts. M4

17. Talking to a friend, a G.P., about his M.E., he commented, " It's like stepping into a different dimension." M4

17. Experiencing strong feelings of being cut off from the light, cut off from love. It's as if I've fallen into a black hole, anti matter, the abyss.

Having a strange feeling that I've done something terribly wrong and was damned. I'd learnt too much and was wrong to want to share this knowledge / wisdom / truth, with the world. It was not my business, only the Gods'. It was up to the Gods' alone to decide our fate, not the domain of a mere mortal. I'd over-stepped my mark. There was no consolation / salvation, not even in death. I feel absolute despair as if my God-Goddess has forsaken me. M4

13. Huge depression over partner, ex of three weeks, also about my son and his chronic illness. My boyfriend betrayed me, I feel. (Got rid of him first week of proving). I don't need to be hurt like this. I've known him since I was a teenager. Love of my life and he is still hurting me (In late fifties now). I hate him and I miss him. M4

13. I've been having suicidal thoughts lately. M4

13. I've been rejecting close relationships now. I don't want anyone to get close to me. I've been crying and crying, crying myself to sleep. M4

14. Fear of having liver or colon cancer. M4

4. Fear of having lung cancer. M4

17. I'm very sensitive to criticism. M4

7. I've been very sensitive to criticism. I had to go outside and pretend to have a cigarette yesterday, when my boss criticised me, as I didn't want him to see my tears. M4

17. Missed my pickup to go singing this evening, by taking a wrong turning and getting jammed in traffic. I sat in my car and felt overwhelmed by sadness. I decided to visit a friend instead, but got halfway there, came to a roundabout at a crossroads and had no idea where I was (on a very familiar stretch of road). It frightened me and I wondered if I was safe to drive.

Then the emotions began to rise again and I broke down and sobbed. I cried and cried, tears springing from the bottom of my heart. M4

17. My heart physically aches. I feel rejected, all alone, unloved. I tried to get on with things but my heart is a leaden weight pulling me down. M4

17. I feel as if I'm pregnant, such a nice feeling, my breasts are enlarged and I don't want to eat rubbish food. M4

7. Feel this remedy has brought my main 'issue' to the fore. My lesson is to learn to let go of emotional pain. M4

17. My mind is racing, but I am unable to calm down and trap ideas on paper.
Sometimes feel that I'm burning up, I've so much nervous energy. M5

17. For months I've felt an underlying unease. Either the world is going to be destroyed or maybe destruction is on personal level. I've become very aware of the conflict between alternative vs. institutional viewpoint, and the risk of harassment to oppose accepted views, e.g. Mr Purdy re. Organo-phosphates. M5

17. Feel as if there is something alive in my abdomen, a huge tapeworm or bilharzia worms. M5

17. While washing my hair in the bath, head under water, had the sensation of being shot. Thought I was getting too close to the truth. This was followed by an image of my partner throwing a plugged-in radio into the bath. Could I not even trust him? M5

12. I feel inadequate as a person. I have to get my relationships with people sorted. M5

12. I've been zooming off into space. M5

12. Having sexual fantasies. M5

12. I'm frightened of contacting people, re: work for fear of being rejected. M5

17.   I'm beginning to seriously question my sanity.  M5

17.   Recurring feeling of being blocked on all levels. I resolve problems but don't seem to move on.   M6

17.   I'm feeling total despair over my current situation, there appears to be no solution. I feel numb. I don't feel. I caught myself thinking of Christ on the cross. How did he feel: " Father, why have you forsaken me?" I know how he felt.   M6

18.   Feel absolute despair. What is the point in anything? Feel numb. I have a beautiful wife, children, set -up, but I can't feel any optimism for it. I'm suicidal, nothing can help me.   M6

7.   Really felt my energy change during an x- ray, after I felt completely wiped out.   M7

17.   I find myself playing the fiddle, the first time for years. I've had such a block. But now I feel confidant and in control. In fact this is how I feel about life in general. Cure?   M7

1.   A lot of people are coming into my space with cancer. I'm learning a lot from them, like how the more spiritually orientated pass on in peace. The materialistic have a harder time, and their families.   M7

10.   I felt such disillusionment in my work; I wanted out and have given in my notice.   M7

10.   Nothing seems to touch me normally. I'm untouched by emotions, although I do feel compassion. Yet, very dramatic things have been thrown up in my life during this proving to jolt me. My emotions have been tested to the limit, losses going on, irritation, anger, annoyance and resentments.   00

10.   I don't feel at all motivated at the moment, yet I've loads to do.  00

10.   Keep finding myself in an ' in between time', a place where time has no value.

Stars, Planets,
Gods of night, pierce the darkness and call to me,
I stare,
On a clear night I can see eternity,
and eternity stares back at me,
bringing me knowledge, helping,
letting me know my strengths, my weaknesses.
And deep inside
I feel you will always be there.    00

17.    Keep finding myself in situations where time appears to stand still. It's as if I step into a gap in time, where time has no value.    00

2.    I'm working with more and more men who are trying to find a new role model for men. Not macho, but what? It is very heartening especially as once again W.W.III hangs over our heads.    00

2.    Feel as if I've got something bad in my body, as if I'm recovering from a bad over dose.    00

2.    This is not reality.    00

2.    Thought I may have cancer of the thymus.    00

2.    Wanted to be at home, doing things at home, nice and quiet.    00

2.    I've been falling asleep whilst listening to dull patients!    00

2.    I've been so busy and so tired; I've had to be very firm, justifiably with my patients and students. I really need space for me.    00

2.    At times I think I'm losing it.    00

2.    I feel deathly tired.    00

2.    I'm going through a life change. I've finished the mother phase and I'm moving on to the next phase. I feel vibrant and much more in my self.. Feel optimistic and positive about my future. I'm organising a party to celebrate and I'm changing my surname.    00

17.    I feel I've left this reality, but haven't reached anywhere else. It's as if I'm in limbo.    00

8.    I'm starting to drift away from this earth and I'm questioning whether I actually want to remain here, or is there a better alternative. I've become tired with the struggles of this life. I no longer have the energy to deal with them.    00

17.    I'd love a rest from the pressures of this world.    00

10,11.    Less mental / emotional symptoms with this proving. Much more a remedy acting on the physical!    00

2.    My brain won't catch up with my head?    00

15.    I've been feeling very angry at my situation at home. I'm rebelling against a situation where I'm always piggy in the middle. I'm bitchy and irritable.    00

15.    Feeling of lack of self-worth and hopelessness. There is no solution to my situation.    00

1.    Feeling of total peace and stillness.    00

17.    I feel this remedy has pushed me beyond my fears and I feel much calmer, more powerful and full of trust in life.    00

9.    Spent the eve of my 40th birthday attending my Uncle's funeral. 00

9.    Found myself talking to my brother-in-law about murder. Someone I know has an ex-boyfriend who has just stabbed someone more than forty times. Then we talked about his brother who had committed suicide 8 years ago. Then we met a friend whose mother had died recently of cancer. All this talk of death, yet there was no sombre feeling or depression, just one of acceptance. Life goes on sort of thing.    00

9.    I'm wondering whether this remedy ties in with Pluto, ruler of the 8th sign Scorpio, death and rebirth.    00

9.    I feel positive, motivated. Secure, self assured, realistic, aware of my needs and limitations.    00

9.    I'm aware of colours. All my senses are heightened.    00

9.     I'm very busy then later I feel very, very tired. I had M.E. some years ago and it reminds me very much of that. It's as if this remedy pushes you to your limit so that you know where it is. It makes you work on yourself, i.e., if you are immensely tired you have to nurture yourself.   00

9.     I'm having moments of intense contentment.   00

2.     As soon as the remedy arrived I felt lousy. I felt tired all the time, but the main impact was psychological.

2.     I feel ratty, impatient and intolerant.   00

2.     I was busy, but no more than I often am, but I really felt like I couldn't cope. I was overloaded. Everything was too much to do, to organise, to be responsible for. I felt overwhelmed. This time it really felt too big a burden for me to hold.   00

2.     I'm finding it hard to separate reality from feelings.   00

2.     I was feeling overwhelmed by my children's needs.   00

2.     I was really pissed off with my clients! I felt distanced, apart somehow. I did not want social contact or any human contact really.   00

2.     I'm feeling so weird.   00

2.     I've been a bit manic, not doing anything well or properly. Rushing around being useless, feeling overwhelmed by everything.   00

2.     I hate my partner; he's being so awful.   00

2.     After Christmas I was really busy, but I coped with it. I paced myself, prioritised. I knew I couldn't keep going at this pace.   00

2.     I felt bizarre, best word I can think of. My thoughts are not in my control.   00

2.     Had a huge outburst of total fury. Had a row with partner, went upstairs because I did not trust myself not to say damaging things. My son got scared as I was crying such a lot. I went over to the barn, where I screamed and raged and generally

had a tantrum. I felt quite scared at the strength of my emotion. My partner came to see if I was OK and I yelled at him, sent him away. We did not speak for several days. I still felt angry and knew I wouldn't be able to communicate rationally. Eventually I rang a co-counsellor. 00

2. I've been having suicidal thoughts and it's really frightening. I've wanted to drive into a lorry, even with my children in the car. 00

2. I'm losing grip on reality, more mental than emotional, fantasies, paranoia, and suicidal thoughts. I'm flipping in and out of reality. Have never experienced these feelings before, I treat people with these. 00

2. I took Lach. 30 c [const.] as an antidote and the suicidal fantasies went. The strong psychological, fantasy, paranoia has gone from the front of my mind but is still lurking somewhere. Fantasies and paranoia mainly around killing myself and my children. 00

2. I feel like I do when I'm pregnant. My body does not want coffee, alcohol or rubbish foods. 00

2. I know that I am well balanced, sensible etc., but I feel strongly that I am losing it at the moment. Is it white coats time? 00

2. I am out of the earth's atmosphere, linking into the beauty of the living earth. 00

2. I've been drawn to wear turquoise to help me ground. 00

2. There is no joy between my partner and I. There is nothing actually wrong, nothing clear, nothing real. 00

# Vertigo

16.  Evening, started to feel very dizzy, not drunk feeling but very uncomfortable. I was quite worried I needed to simply sit. Very, very strong feeling, not pleasant, lasted approx. $^1/_2$ hr.  D-5

5.  Head felt spinney. 1$^{st}$ few mins

16.  Strong dizziness, a definite feeling that I could not drive the car. Machines felt out of my control, wanted to go nowhere near them.  D1

10.  Late afternoon and early evening slight sensation of vertigo, lasting only a split second. Mother-in-law is also suffering from vertigo at the moment and husband complained of it a few days ago.  D3

5.  Morning felt very dizzy, was sick and had diarrhoea.  D4

5.  My head feels spinney when I grab some college work or a book. A feeling of brain overload.  D6

13.  While walking to school - dizzy spells. It was awful; I was frightened to speed up in case I fainted. Felt like I was going to collapse. Brought with it a fear of heart problems.  D27

15.  Experienced vertigo while lying down and when looking up - loss of balance.  M3

Gen.

[5,11,8,4,13, Vertigo-dizziness,
10,17,15]
[17,11,4,8,5.]    -on rising.  M3

# Head

| 5,17. | Feels as if temples are depressed. D1 |
|---|---|

5,17.     Feels as if temples are depressed. D1

10.     Scalp feels tingly. D1

9.     Slight headache. D1

10.     Woke feeling tired with a congested headache, mouth fill of clear phlegm. Headache left side extending to left back teeth. Found it difficult to get things together for breakfast, just wanted to go back to bed and rest. D2

5.     Head felt constricted during evening. D2

12.     Slight congestion of head and runny nose. D2

16.     Head feels heavy. D5

8.     Head full of catarrh today. D6

7.     Slight tension type headache, with tension in neck and shoulders. Neck and shoulders feel crunchy. D7

8.     Got the beginning of a headache, so I decided to inhale with Eucalyptus oil!!! It had worked before. However, the smell was too strong for me to cope with. I felt overwhelmed by the vapours and it hurt my nasal passages and eyes. D10

17.     Itchy head feels as if I've got nits. D12

17.     Looks as if my hair is thinning above the temples. M2

17.     Woke into slight frontal headache, sinus area. Hung around for days. M2

17.     Headache, dreadful migraine. Seems to be a blocked sinus variety, frontal, forehead pounding. It feels as if there is an immense pressure deep inside my head, in my inner sanctum. I had to lie down, as the pain was overwhelming. With it photophobia and nausea. M2

8.     Head felt heavy and drowsy and I longed for fresh air. M3

8.     Woke up and head was thumping. It was extremely difficult walking up and down stairs. I was better moving around, rather

than sitting still. It was agony getting up and down. Felt close to tears several times. I longed for fresh air, but it was still raining. I had a raging temperature. M3

8. Woke feeling better but head is 'muzzy'. M3

17. Chronic itchy head, and with it a feeling of being uncomfortable in my body. M4

8. My brain hurts. I feel dehydrated as if my brain is shrinking, drawing away from inside my skull. Is this what alcoholics feel like? M4

4. Headache in forehead and left temple. Forehead felt hot. I felt generally feverish and very tired. M4

17. Heat in head, particularly my forehead, which feels very hot to touch. M5

5,8,17. Head feels blocked with catarrh. M5

7. Woke into pounding headache with raging temperature and feeling dehydrated. M5

17. Eruptions on hairline, which are itchy but don't develop. 00

8. Itchy little eruptions, hairline. Previously connected with stress. 00

2. I've had more headaches than I've ever had in my life. Headache located at two points on the top of my head, extending up from my eyes. My eyes hurt and I can't concentrate. 00

15. Thumping headache. Congested head with stuffed up nose and earache. Feverish. 00

17. Headache forehead and left temple. Felt like pressure from within. 00

2. Headache like a pressure from inside my head, mainly behind forehead and lt. Temple. 00

8. Have had a slight headache for days, wake with it. Around front of head and sinus area. 00

# Eyes - Vision

17. The world around me has come into focus. Colours are brighter, more vivid and objects more crisp / clearly defined.    D1

16. Eyes are looking bloodshot.    D1

Gen.
[5,7,17, 8,14,10.]    Eyes feel heavy.    D1

12. Heightened clarity of vision. In focus, colours bright, image clear.    D2

16. Colours appear stronger today, very bright, very noticeable. Like a dust has been washed off the lenses of the eye.    D2

10. Eyes felt hot in morning on waking.    D10

8. Eyes are dry and itchy.    M1

17. Eyes look sunken.    M1

17. My eyes feel dry and itchy, as if foreign body or dust in them. I rub them and they become sore.    M2

Gen.
[10,1,8, 7,17,5.]    Itchy eyes.    M2

8. My eyes felt as if they were sinking into the back of my skull. M4

2. Can't focus my eyes. They ache and I've become photophobic. I'm having to wear sunglasses. 00

17. I've got tired eyes. 00

2. I've got bags under my eyes. (? kidneys low) 00

# Ears - Hearing

8.      I've a high-pitched whine in my ears.   D2

17.     High pitched buzzing in my ears.   D3

1.      Earache - concomitant of infected gum. Ears are buzzing, a high-pitched noise.   D8

7.      Scabby bits in both ears that remain wet and don't heal properly. I keep picking at them, slightly itchy.   M2

8.      Left ear blocked. Finding it difficult to hear. Mucous in Eustachian tube. Painless, but with it a sore throat, like razor blades. Blew my nose and it cleared my tube, hearing fine now.   M4

17.     Had a fly in my ear!   00

8,17.   Sharp pain in left Ear.   00

15.     Earache with congested head, stuffed up nose. Thumping headache. Feverish.   00

# Nose

## Gen.

[5,8,7,17, 10,1,14.] Nose feels sore as if with a cold.   First $\frac{1}{2}$ hr.

12.       Runny nose, watery discharge.   D2

17.       Nose uncomfortable, dry inside. Rubbing my nose and picking. Very aware of my nose (merc.)   D2

17.       Woke up with blocked nose and sinus. I can't smell. Much catarrh, hawking solid lumps. Initial lump this morning very smelly, almost putrid. At first greenish / yellow then white through to clear. After the solid lump the discharge went from stringy to loose. With it a pressure behind my forehead and behind my eyes, with a high pitched buzzing in my ear. (All the family is suffering with catarrh at the moment.)

Note: Connection with disordered digestive system and catarrh. Catarrh = toxins being expelled from body, if digestive system is not efficient.   D3

8.        I'm full of catarrh today.   D8

10.       Sneezing lots during evening, followed by running nose, clear. Did not interfere with my breathing.   D8

10.       Nose running in evening and first thing in the morning.   D9

8.        Nose running like a tap, a clear discharge.   D9

8.        Very aware of smells. I think my sinuses are clearer than they've been for a long time.   D11

7.        My sinuses feel clear, first time for ages.   M1

17,7.     Increased mucous in morning.   M1

7.        Waking up with blocked nose, as I get going it begins to clear. Mainly sinus clearing. Discharge yellow / greenish.   M1

17.       Left nostril sore.   M2

7.        Nose dry and uncomfortable. Left nostril sore to touch.   M2

8.   Pick it and it bleeds. Scabs over, and I pick it again. It feels dry and horrid, worse in the morning. M2

7.   Picking at scabby bits in my nose. M2

11.  Bouts of violent sneezing. M2

17.  My sinuses have finally cleared. M2

17.  My son had a nosebleed. M2

8.   I had a nosebleed. M3

11.  Cold came out of the blue, not even a sore throat to warn me. Total head cold. Nose running like a tap. Clear discharge. With it a desire to drink lots of water. Felt like an instant detox. M3

7.   Have increased catarrh. Blocked nose and I can't smell. With it a pressure behind my eyes and in forehead. 00

17.  A fly flew up my nose! 00

8.   Blocked nose extending to sinus. Pressure behind my eyes and forehead. I've a lot of catarrh at the moment, thick yellow discharge. 00

7.   I can't stand the smell of coffee, alcohol or tobacco smoke. I'm very sensitive to smells now. M7

# Face

10.    Feeling of energy in upper cheeks, as if I'd been laughing a lot. Look red and jolly. First $1/2$ hr.

Gen.    Cheek bones ache. As if been chewing gum or laughing a lot.
[1,7,17,    D1
8,5,14.]

1.    Hot flushes, face looks blood red.  D2

17.    Tension around lower jaw and cheekbone, ext. to neck.  D3

8.    Spots on face. Hormonal?  D28

14.    Two bouts of pimples on my face, before and after my period. Crap coming out.  M1

17.    Face flushed, due to increased body heat.  M3

11.    Pussy spots on face and an eczema type rash on forehead, red itchy and raised.  M3

2.    Massive outbreak of ringworm on face, beginning left cheek extending to right.  00

17, 4.    Face looks drawn.  M3

17.    Look pale and anaemic.  M4

17.    My son has developed dry red patches on face, around nose, cheeks, upper and lower lips and chin. Reacted to all creams, except one with entirely natural ingredients.  00

# Mouth - Teeth

8.    Mouth ulcers, sore mouth inside. 00

1.    Broke two teeth left side. Became infected and lasted a week. Very painful shooting pains radiating to ears with earache and a high-pitched noise. Massive cold sore, left side. Then got flu. D8

8,12,17.    Dry mouth. Loss of taste. 00

Gen.
[5,7,1,8, 17.]    Sensitive teeth. M3

17.    Incisor upper left {previous sight of abscess} is painful, as if pressure building up inside. M3

Gen.
[10,8, 17,4.]    Grinding teeth in bed at night. M3

17.    Sore mouth inside as if about to produce mouth ulcers. M3

12.    My mouth is sore inside, as if I'd had salt in mouth. Feels as if it may form ulcers. M3

1.    Abscess of tooth, upper incisor. 00

18.    False tooth on pin, fell out. Nasty taste in mouth, of decay. Gums bleeding. M4

4.    Have ground my teeth down to the pulpy bits in the middle. M4

5.    Sensitive teeth and a loose tooth. M4

2.    Visit to dentist, she says I have more of a reaction to the amount of plaque than would normally be expected. 00

17.    Swallowed a fly. 00

17.    Grinding teeth during day. 00

# Throat

**Gen.**

[7,5,14, 17,1,8,10.]     Dry throat, slightly sore. First $^1/_2$ hr.

10.     Lots of phlegm in throat. First $^1/_2$ hr.

10.     Sore throat on waking, coughed up red / brown sputum. D7

10.     Throat felt congested, on waking. D10

4.     Sore dry throat. Catarrh and discomfort in throat and upper chest. These are symptoms I had a year ago, when I had M.E. D17.

7.     Coughing up greenish sputum, particularly bad in the morning on waking, occasionally flecked with black. Feel as if my lungs are having a good clear out. M3

17.     Coughing up salty / cheesy tasting mucus, worse morning on waking, white / thick at first becoming clear. Last night woke at 3am and hawked up a thick yellowy lump. Feel this is a needy clear out of my lungs. M4

## Throat ext.

17.     Glands (cervical) in my neck slightly swollen, sore to touch. Skin feels irritated, tight over thyroid. Slightly numb sensation right side. Have a floating lump-flat, size of Soya bean right of thyroid. M4

2.     My thyroid feels tight, which would account for my tiredness; this constant feeling of having a hangover. Waking up feeling tired and listless. 00

5.     Aware of my thyroid at the moment. 00

2.     Painful swollen glands - cervical. 00

# Stomach

1.     Indigestion- stomach / abdomen is bubbling. First ¹/₂ hr.

10.    Incarcerated wind in upper chest, feel the need to belch. Not better for belching. First ¹/₂ hr.

17.    Stomach feels uncomfortable, sort of indigestion. Slight nausea, with sickly burps, which afford no relief. First ¹/₂ hr.

5.     My 3 year old son who was present but in another room was sick. He was good-humoured about it, no distress. First ¹/₂ hr.

10.    Nausea with sick-like burps, which did not relieve. Felt I needed to eat something. D1

4.     Hiccoughs when taking remedy and hiccoughs at bedtime. Found it hard to get rid of them. D1

5.     Woke up this morning feeling nauseous. Had to get up and be sick. Suffered nausea and vomiting most of the day. The vomit was yellow and tasted sweet. D4

8.     Felt sick most of morning and didn't eat until 11.45am. D5

8.     Acute indigestion- experiencing nausea especially after eating. Stomach gurgling and I'm burping loudly. Hot feeling inside and up into my throat. Odd sharp pains in abdomen above hips. Stomach, just below sternum painful when I gently press. Feel out of sorts. D10

8.     Plagued by nausea and it hurt when I breathed, following a reaction to exhaust fumes earlier in the day. D11

17.    Stomach feels bloated and uncomfortable, yet I'm not over eating. D11

17.    Feel a heat in stomach as if it's on fire. Top of legs are burning. D14

5.     My 2 year old son suffered a bout of nausea and vomiting. No fever- no real distress. Maybe aggravated by mixed foods earlier. Fine within an hour and eating again. D11

17.    Feeling nauseous which is slightly amel. after eating. D21

17. Burning thirst. M1

17,10. Slight nausea for weeks. 00

7. Really noisy stomach, especially in bed. M1

9. Boil on solar plexus - doesn't feel like it will come to anything. M1

8. I've been feeling nauseous for weeks. When the nausea stopped I began to suffer sharp pains under my breastbone. M2

8. Bloated stomach although I'm not overeating. It feels really uncomfortable if I do. M2

1. My stomach has been really bloated as if I'm pregnant. It's very uncomfortable yet I haven't eaten much. 00

7. Bloated stomach, hard and very uncomfortable. No great appetite. 00

17. Have lost my appetite. M2

7. Have no hunger when I wake. M2

8. During the afternoon felt very nauseous. Headache brewing. Stomach gurgling and rumbling. Ate nothing till 7.30 p.m. Next day woke up still feeling nauseous with a raging temperature. M2

17. Lost my sense of taste. M3

17. Stomach feels blocked, bloated - full of wind, gurgling. I feel pregnant when I bend forward. M5

7. Pain, incredibly tender in stomach. Can't move, it's too painful. With it a slight nausea and a raging temperature. M7

# Abdomen

17. Immediately on taking the remedy experienced feeling of discomfort in region of liver.

1. Much bubbling in my abdomen and much more flatulence than normal. D1

17. During ultra sound investigation a polyp / calculus was noticed in my gall bladder. No thickening of the wall. I've had no symptoms to suggest such. D3

5. Around 2 am - tight, constricting pains in upper and lower abdomen. Slight relief if I put pressure on solar plexus area. Very uncomfortable, didn't sleep much. D3

1. My kidney and gall bladder area aches, a dull ache. My stomach is bloated. D5

7. Abdomen is bubbling and with it a lot of flatulence. D7

17. Abdomen {transverse colon} and stomach {epigastrium} are bubbling / fermenting. D7

8. Abdomen is bubbling; with it increased flatus. 00

1. Felt pains in right side of my waist and under right ribs, in region of gall bladder. {Had a cholecystectomy 8 yrs ago} Stabbing stitching pains. Can't bear anything around my waist. I think I'm going to cut out fats. The glands at the inner top of my legs are sore and swollen. D7

7. Bloated abdomen, feels uncomfortable. D11

8. Odd sharp pains in abdomen above hips. D11

4. Pain in right groin. Same pain as I had years ago linked with Irritable bowel syndrome (IBS) a sharp stabbing pain. D14

8. My glands are up in my right inner thigh, slightly sore and swollen. D14

17. Right inguinal nodes are sore to touch and slightly swollen. D14

17.     Pains in right hypochondrium / liver - goes from stabbing, stitching to drawing, aching. With it a bubbling sensation. This region feels hot inflamed, congested and full. Last night's indulgence with alcohol and tobacco has aggravated. I can't take pressure of clothes around my waist, in fact I don't want anyone to touch me, it might hurt. The pains are agg. by bending forward, squatting, driving, getting cold and any exertion. These symptoms were noticeably agg. after a highly emotional episode / argument with my partner. I can't sleep knee to chest in bed as this agg, within mins. D15

8.     Sharp pain opposite side to my appendix. I felt a lump of gas / wind, which dispersed after rubbing. M2

8.     Cramping pain in abdomen and stomach. M2

11.     Have been aware of my spleen- feeling of sensitivity in this area, reminiscent of 18 months ago when I suffered a burst spleen- saved by a wizard surgeon. Spleen had been swollen due to flu and I'd knocked it accidentally. M2

7.     Had colicky pains in abdomen- doubled up in pain. I then had diarrhoea and felt better. M2

17.     Feeling of heat in abdomen. M2

17.     Noticed a lump in abdomen left side, after rubbing it dispersed, just blocked gas. M2

17.     Pain in right hypochondrium, occasionally extending to iliac fossa. Hot, sharp pains. I began to fear my appendix would burst. Sharp pain under

ribs right up through into bottom of lung, extending to right lower scapula. M2

8.     Stitching pain all around my midriff. M3

8.     Ache and sensitivity around my waist. M3

1.     Sharp pain, acute, unbearable under ribs right I had to go outside and walk around until it abated. M3

17.     Stitching pain in right and left hypochondrium, under ribs.

I'm familiar now with the right sided pain. But this has now extended to left (spleen / pancreas?) This whole area (solar plexus) feels vulnerable. I don't want anyone near. It's aggravated by any pressure. M3

1.   Stitching pain in region of groin right   M3

10.  Feel a weakness in upper abdomen.   00

17.  Last night as I lay on my back in bed, experienced sharp pain in what I imagined to be my spleen. I became quite perturbed, thinking the pain would get worse and my spleen would burst. I might die. Hot, inflamed all around waist, my hottie agg. this.   M3

17.  Feeling bruised now that intense pain has gone from left and right hypochondrium. Left side feels weak.   M4

17.  Abdomen feels blocked, bloated, windy, gurgling. Feels as if there is something alive in there, a tapeworm or bilharzia worms.   M5

7.   Incredible tender pain in abdomen agg. by any movement. With it a raging temp.   M7

17.  Pelvic bone aches, feels stiff, as if I've been sitting for too long. Is better for walking although stiff at first. But gets stiff again after walking for a while. I feel dragged down and have to sit.   M4

# Rectum

1. Had an accident. Thought I'd farted but that was not all! First ¹/₂ hr.

7. Itchy anus, which is worse at night and in bed.  D2

5. Morning- felt dizzy was sick and had diarrhoea, at first watery stools no solids at all. Then stools turned yellow. Sick also yellow and tasted sweet. Passed out for a few moments. Moved from bed to toilet all day. Felt weak. No food all day, just sips of water.  D4

17. Itchy bum, as if I have worms.  D5

17. Sore anus.  D5

10. Itchy bum and more wind than normal.  D7

1. More flatulence than normal and a sore anus.  D7

17. Increased flatus, not always offensive.  D7

17. Blind boil in crack of bum right side.  Sore to touch and when sitting. Hot to touch. (Didn't resolve )  D8

1. Flatus feels stuck, incarcerated.  D11

8. Have been constipated over the last few days, it's easing gradually, but I'm still not regular.  D11

17. Uncontrollable diarrhoea for two days, then intermittent over seven days. Diarrhoea at first watery moving to loose yellow. D14

10. Making more trips to the loo. Bowels never feel completely empty.  D21

17. Bowel movement more frequent. Unsatisfactory stool - unfinished.  D21

10. Constipation for two days.  D28

8. Itchy anus as if have worms.  M2

8. Have been getting diarrhoea twice a day. Urgency, have no choice but to go.  M2

1. Diarrhoea- have to go. Have occasionally misjudged and have had an accident. 00

11. Going to the loo more, stools slightly loose. M2

7. I've been feeling heavy and sluggish, particularly after eating meat.Became constipated for two days. Then colicky pains in abdomen. I was doubled up in pain. I then had diarrhoea, which relieved the pain. M2

7. Been getting boils on my bum that don't happen. Raised, red and sore but never progress and resolve. M2

8. Loose stools for weeks but now I've been constipated for three days. With it increased flatulence, which smells of faeces. M2

8,7,17,1. Flatus, Sometimes with slight discharge for weeks. Mostly odourless. M2

17. Desire to go to the loo often, but empty. 00

13. I'm having too many bowel movements. M3

13. Bowels never feel completely empty. M3

17. Have been constipated but not uncomfortable. M3

# Stool

1.     Involuntary stools - painless.  D2

5.     Stools watery at first with no solids, then becoming yellow.  D4

17.    Involuntary stools, painless. Loose and watery, sometimes pungent - putrid. Excoriating. Becoming soft, yellow stools.  D14

8.     Loose stools for weeks.  M2

# Urinary Organs

## Bladder / Urine

1. Increased desire to urinate. D1

17. Urine smells strong, not offensive? Sweet. Slightly excoriating, as if getting cystitis, plus a dragging down feeling. D5

17. Wee strong yellow in colour. D16

17. Having to wee more often. D21

10. Needing to wee more often. D25

11. I've been peeing a lot more than usual. M2

17. Excoriating urine -? Cystitis threatening. Urine smells strong, between sweet and sulphurous. M3

# Kidneys

1. My kidneys ache, a dull ache. D4

17. Kidneys feel inflamed. Area hot to touch. M2

# Female Genitalia

17.  Itchy labia - external.  D1

10.  Started my period today at 4pm, this is really unusual as I normally start at 8am. Otherwise normal.  D5

10.  Period seems to have stopped completely - very unusual, normally would have stopped tomorrow.  D7

17.  Finally rid of pubic itch.  D8

17.  Slight vaginal discharge, creamy, not smelly.  D10

15.  Intolerable itch, mons pubis, region of hair only.  00

17.  Uterine pain, like a period pain and bloating. Worse for a hot bath.  D21

12.  Congested feeling in womb and a period pain, although I'm not on.  D26

17.  Boil just behind labia right. Not coming to a head. Whole area is sore and slightly swollen.  D28

2.  Dry itch around vagina - labia. Like thrush but without a discharge.  00

8,7,17,10.  Menses late.  M2

11.  Missed a period this month, just a tiny bit of spotting. Grumbly aches in ovaries.  M2

7.  Period at moment - day two felt nauseous all day.  M2

7.  Have thrush, sore and itchy. No discharge. Worse at night in bed, preventing sleep. Red raw and swollen. I can't stop myself from scratching it, from    pudenda to anus.  M2

4.  When my back felt well enough, we resumed sexual relations {1st time in a year or 2} my back immediately felt worse again. Also experiencing pain in vagina, when it contracts during orgasm, it hurts. Trying to tell myself this is scar tissue, but deep down find the whole thing sickeningly worrying. Since my sex life doesn't look hopeful I can ignore it.  M2

15. Maddening itch on pudenda. I've scratched so much I've got bald patches, literally pulled my hair out. It's worse at night in bed, when heated. Tried fungal creams to no avail.  M2

2. Have been off sex for months, but my libido has now returned.  M2

17. My libido is good at the moment. I've had a sudden surge and realised that it's been non-existent for months.  M2

17. Clear discharge, slightly smelly - cheesy.  M2

11. Normal period this month, but now 2 weeks later already spotting, accompanied by abdominal pain.  M3

17. Sore, itchy labia and surrounding area. As if getting thrush, but no discharge.  M4

17. Breasts enlarged run up to menses and remained for a week after. Sore to touch, as if I was pregnant.  M4

11. Feel pre-period, although I've just had one.  M4

1. Rash which looks like ringworm in groin, moving towards labia. Red whelks x 2, one the size of a penny, the other $\frac{1}{2}$ penny. Very itchy. Sometimes stings. Tight trousers agg. It's been on and off for months.  M8

# Respiration

## Gen.

[7,5,14, 10,1,8,17.] Breathless. First ¹/₂ hr.

8.      I'm having to consciously take a breath. First ¹/₂ hr.

9.      I'm breathing deep (normally shallow). D7

8.      Noticing exhaust fumes lately. Aware of breathing them in, making my chest feel tight. I felt poisoned by them, as if they were infiltrating my body, down my tubes, into my lungs, spreading across my chest. I wanted to breathe fresh clean air. Later I was plagued by nausea and it hurt when I breathed out. D11

17.     Have felt a marked sensitivity to chemicals - paint, petrol, farmer's sprays, even the smell of silage. Neighbouring farmer has sprayed today and initially I experienced a burning in nose, throat and top of chest. Followed by a headache in forehead and left temple. Forehead became hot and I felt feverish, my energy sunk within hours. It felt like a return of my M.E. symptoms.

        Last week I stripped a wood panel of paint and I felt ill for a week. I go from nervous/restless energy to absolute fatigue. Accompanied by aches and sensitivity around upper waist {liver, colon, and spleen?}. D12

17.     Can't get a full lung of air due to pain and bloatedness of epigastrium. D21

13.     Short of breath walking to school. Shallow breathing. D27

17.     Lots of mucous in upper respiratory tract in morning, causing a slight wheeze on inspiration. M2

4.      Felt as if I had a chest infection or cold coming. Burning sensation down into top of chest and throat. With headache in forehead and left temple. Forehead hot, I felt feverish and very tired. M4

15.   Chest infection, coughing up green sputum, which goes to clear.
00

7.   Chest infection - coughing up green sputum.   M7

# Chest

7.    Palpitations as if in panic or excitement.  1$^{st}$ $^1/_2$ hr

8.    Warm panicky feeling from heart centre, but no palpitations. 1$^{st}$ $^1/_2$ hr

8,17.  Heartburn.  1$^{st}$ $^1/_2$ hr

4.    Prickling / itching sensation over ribs, felt like shingles.  D1

8.    During evening experienced fluttering in chest / heart area. Still felt unbalanced.  D3

17.   Ache in heart.  D3

17.   Stitching pain in heart radiating left  D4

8.    Strange sensations in left breast after activity.  D26

8.    Sharp pain under breastbone.  M1

2.    Eruption red raised in middle of sternum.  00

14.   Bruised feeling under right rib cage, in the area of my gall bladder.  M1

17.   Cramping pain under rib cage - epigastrium extending right M1

8.    Woke several times in night with soreness in left breast. In morning woke with more tenderness in left breast.  M2

17.   Extreme sensitivity and prickling sensation around my lower ribs, mainly front and sides. Extending to liver, which feels hot. Can't wear anything around my waist. I've noticed it's worse before emptying my bowels and slightly relieved after. Worse lying on back and worse lying with right knee up to chest or lying right side. This can extend to pelvic girdle as a strange ache / sensitivity.  M2

17.   Burning sensation under ribs and breastbone. Dull ache in breastbone, sore to touch.  M2

8. Really hurting beneath breastbone, a dull ache. I've been feeling nauseous for weeks, when nausea stopped began to suffer with sharp pains under breastbone. M2

7. Lump in breast, very tender. M3

17. Heart racing, uncontrollable palpitations even when lying down. After exercise my heart would not return to normal rate. M3

7. I have developed shingles. Started with a few itchy spots on left side of chest and slowly spread to right side of chest. This whole area is extremely sensitive to touch. I can't stand anything around my waist. With it a feeling of being worn down. I'm so tired at the moment. M3

17. Severe pain under ribs right as if a knife was stuck up under rib cage. Radiating to iliac fossa. With a slight temp, feel chilly. Pain agg. lying on rt. side. Waist feels sore. M3

17. Eruption, red raised and inflamed in middle of sternum {thymus?}. This was the final site of an all over body rash I had for a year as a child, after swimming in the sea which had allegedly been contaminated by mustard gas. M3

5. Pain in chest at heart level. Incredibly tender, very painful when moving, walking. M7

# Back

16. Strange ache across shoulders, more like carrying the head in a really conscious way. Felt myself pulling and stretching shoulder muscles.  PP D-3

10,1. Chilly, shivery feeling up back, between shoulder blades.  1st ½ hr.

8. Painful neck and shoulders have gone since taking the Rx. {curative}  D2

8. Painful neck and shoulders have returned after big emotional crisis in current relationship. Pain is on right side, which is achy and stiff.  D3

9. Back is aching, painful, and stiff.  D3

17. Pain under lower right scapula, extending into right shoulder joint. Like a knot of tension. Painful for pressure, better rubbing. Assoc. with pain under right rib cage, front and biliary colic type symptoms.  D4

7. Neck has been aching a bit, feels stiff. I have a crunchy neck, feels tense, with a slight tension headache. Worse for the cold, damp, wet weather.  D7

4. Lent forward to open gate from back of horse. Gate was heavier than I'd expected. Unpleasant, though not painful sensation in my back.  D8

4. Pulled my back wrestling with a drawer, then bent over to pick something up and felt the most excruciating pain in lower right back. Legs went wobbly and kept collapsing. Felt sick. Saw Reflexologist / Masseur, who told me it was the muscle in my middle lower back that is affected, and the pain I feel is referred pain.  D9

4. Still cannot walk more than a few yards. I'm doubled over, using a stick to support myself.  D10

4.     No back pain on waking. Walked dogs a short way. By late afternoon, toothache like pain in lower right hip. Muscles in legs trembling. D15

13.    Crunchy shoulders, mainly left. D27

14.    I have a frozen left shoulder, which feels hard and stiff. With it a bruised feeling under right rib cage, in the area of my gall bladder. M1

17.    Ache in shoulder joint right side. Pain is boring, rheumatic, feels stiff. Sometimes it crunches. It hurts to pull my jumper over my head. It is restricting my movement. I feel a sharp pain if I try to move against the stiffness. M2

10.    Aching, boring pain just below left shoulder joint. I feel it if I make a big movement with my arm, but not little movements. It's worse for pressure. Generally feels stiff. M2

8.     Late evening, sharp pain in neck and shoulder right side. M2

7.     Strange pain in head and back, intermittent. Very unpleasant, like a pressure. M2

12.    Burning sensation on back of neck. M2

4.     Pain in back which moves around, sacral mostly also lumbar. Lower part of spine left feels bruised. M2

4.     Pain in back, right lower, agg. coition. M2

17.    Back ache in sacrum and lumbar region, gnawing ache; helped by my hottie (hot water bottle). M2

1.     Back ache in lower back. M3

1.     Ache in pelvis right side, also stitching pains in this region. M3

17.    Stiffness and soreness in back of neck, extending to right shoulder blade. My neck is crunchy and cracks on certain movements. M4

2. The back of my neck aches, it feels tight and tense, like a strain. Sometimes this is accompanied by a headache, a dull ache. Always accompanied by slightly swollen glands in my neck. M5

8. Back ache, particularly lower, lumbar / sacrum, dragging ache. 00

8. Neck, particularly right side stiff and aching, extending to shoulders. Tension. 00

2. Shivery sensation down back of neck and spine. 00

# Extremities

7.      My right knee gave way.  D1

4.      Sore gland in right armpit, reminding me of the M.E. I had last year.  D1

4.      Prickling / itching sensation in my legs.  D1

13.     My hips ache.  D1

12.     Limbs feel stiff and tired.  D2

10.     Hands covered with contact dermatitis, after cutting trees and getting scratched. They are now itchy and spotty. Mid morning left hand, thumb and fingertips were throbbing / tingling, almost numb; as if circulation had gone. This lasted about three minutes.  D2

10.     Hands really itchy and red. Woke up with them driving me mad.  D3

10.     Woke up 4 times during the night scratching my hands. The itching gets really bad with heat. They are extremely spotty and irritable. Itching not bad during the day, but in the evening they become itchy.  D4

1.      My hips feel stiff and achy in the joint. Also my elbow joint. Both are better for heat and exercise.  D4

8,1,17.  Neuralgic pain in lower right hip.   00

8.      Legs aching, knees and soles of feet.  D5

8.      Toes of both feet were itchy and spotty this morning. Lumpy rash, hot red dots under the skin.  D6

10.     Hands still red, itchy, spotty. Put a mix of cham., hyper. and calend. oils on, which does seem to ease it. Have had to take off my wedding ring as the spots have got under it. Finger is slightly swollen.  D6

10.     Only woke twice in the night with my hands. They are still spotty, but not so red and angry, not so itchy.  D7

1.      The glands of my inner legs are sore and swollen.   D7

17.     Aching, drawing pain in wrists, knuckles, knees, ankles, soles
        of feet, shins and thighs. The soles of my feet are sore. It's as
        if I've just walked 300 miles.   D7

1.      Ache in wrists.   D7

Gen.

[8,7,1,17]   Hips ache.   D7

10.     Last night put tiger balm on hands, felt really good and cooling,
        more effective than cham. mix.   D9

10.     Hands are still itchy but are now turning dry in most places.
        D10

17.     Wedding finger is bruised under the ring and slightly swollen.
        I've had to take my ring off, as it's uncomfortable, worse at
        night.   D14

17.     Feet aching, part. ankles joints and toes. Ankles slightly
        swollen, oedematous. Sore to touch. Legs feel heavy and tired,
        with a dragging ache. As if I'd walked for miles. Yet I've been
        inside for days, with no exercise. Burning sensation top of
        legs and heat in stomach. Slight oedematous swelling of knees.
        Ache in right wrist as if strained, worse certain movements
        and applied force.   D14 Repeated M3

17.     By the time I reached my bed, my legs felt almost paralysed.
        I'd had a hot bath which agg. I was concerned that they might
        get worse during the night.   D15

4.      Muscles in legs trembling.   D15

4.      Arms ache badly, upper arm. As if I'd been punched in the
        arm. (This was a symptom of my M.E. last year.)   D16

12.     Left thumb painful. More muscular than joint or bone. Worse
        any pressure. Pain becomes unbearable. Can't move it past a
        point. At rest a pulling pain, like a muscle pull or strain.
        Combined with no strength in hand.   D20

17.     Ache in upper right arm, old vaccination sight.   00

17. Middle finger of right hand feels numb. Finger joints feel stiff and swollen. 00

13. Right hip gave out. Nothing works to help. It won't move. Feels like much too big a space between bones. Won't take any weight. AGONY. Have to drag leg along. It's not going to hold me. Episode lasted $1/2$ hr. I've bought a walking stick. (Major agg. of provers symptoms. This prover has been diagnosed with osteo-arthritic hips. X-rays taken before and after the provings showed an improvement. The hips looked as if they were repairing, which puzzled the doctor! ) D23

13. Left lower thumb joint is stiff. D23

13. Hands very painful ache. Knuckle joints, finger joints and phalanges ache. Burning pain in left knuckle. 1st. finger and sometimes middle finger left almost goes numb and stiff or gets very painful. Difficult to move. Hands feel hot, though not hot to touch. D26

12. Knee hurting, dragging ache. Can't keep my legs still, fidgety. D26

12. Lumps like ganglions on right wrist. Pain in both wrists. Right thumb swollen. Middle finger right swollen. D27

13. Arthritic pains in wrist joints, both hips, fingers and sometimes knees and joint of lt. thumb. Violent, sharp, nasty pain in lt. elbow. Crunchy shoulders mainly left. D27

17. Have a dragging ache in my knees. I've had fidgety legs all day, just can't keep them still. D28

12. Legs feel as if I'd walked for days, so tired. Yet, I've not been at all active. D28

8. Incredibly itchy arms on and of for last two days. D28

4. My legs feel so tired. On going to bed I wondered if I'd wake to find myself paralysed. 00

14. Incredible sensitivity down both legs, which is agg. touching. (Had shingles way back, feels the same.) D30

8.      Legs ache, knees and soles of feet.  M2

8.      Developed a pain in the top of my leg, as if I'd pulled or torn something. The area affected was the top of my thigh, near my pant line, directly in line with my hipbone. I don't remember hurting it and wonder if there is a gland there that might be swollen. The pain prevented me from walking any distance. M2

11.     My right elbow feels 'rheumaticy', stiff and achy.  M2

16.     Eczema type rash on inner thighs, red and itchy, slightly raised. M2

10.     Friction burn on left wrist and three knuckles, minus knuckle of little finger and elbow. Upper left arm ached. Has been developing over days. Now wrist is very, very tender / sore, agg. touch. It's pulsating, very tight and swollen. There is a red line radiating from injury on my wrist, up the vein a 1/3$^{rd}$. of the way up my arm, which feels bruised. Had a big scab, which I lifted to get to the heart of the infection. Under scab white raw flesh, quite deep, developing plasma. Discharge was clear, no pus. It had gone deeper into the blood. Feels slightly neuralgic, as if nerve inflamed.  M3

1.      Stitching pain in my arms.  M3

17.     Cold feet, sometimes icy, as if there is no circulation.  M3

17      Cold numbness in hands and lower arms.  M3

11.     Flu - like aching in my joints and neck.  M3

13.     Pain in right hip, as if running down a ribbon.  M3

13.     My hips are fine.  M4 (Curative ref. D26)

8,17.   Shoulder right aches, stiff. Sharp pains if move against the stiffness. Better heat, locally.  00

8.      Feel strain / sprain in shoulders and arms, down to fingertips; and all through body.  00

8.      Sore gland in right armpit.  00

13. When approx.4 yrs. old I had measles and chickenpox at the same time. Iwas very ill; high fever, pains in legs, drawing ache. Have had pains in legs ever since. At 15/16 yrs. was put on a very strong dose of ?? for severe rheumatism and rheumatoid arthritis, for the pains in my legs. After the proving the pains have gone. M5

10. Have been using heavy chemicals, bleach, and fungicides at work, and this has agg. my hands. M6

10. Wore some new shoes and rubbed my heel. Had to use a plaster although I know I'm allergic to plasters. When I returned home I immediately soaked my foot in lavender. Next day irritating itch where plaster had been; I scratched it a lot. Following day, huge blister had formed on my heal, plus a satellite blister, so I had blisters either side of my heal. They burst and reformed and would burst again. They were filled with yellow odourless pus. They wept constantly. This went on for a week. It didn't itch, wasn't sore. Looked dreadful.

I decided to use Aloe Vera, and then the skin below the blisters became white, waterlogged skin, forming great ridges. The skin had formed honeycombed ridges filled with pus, which smelt sickly sweet, not a familiar smell. Foot healed remarkably well after using Aloe Vera. I'd expected it to last for months. M6

# Sleep

10.     Felt tired earlier than normal, went to bed shattered. D1

17, 10.   Yawning frequently. D1

10.     Woke feeling tired with a congested headache. D2

12.     Not sleeping well, tossing and turning. Body restless, mind busy. D2

1.      Sat down and fell asleep, spilt the drink in my hand. Woke up to a strange smell, like ether. D2

12.     Although I'm extremely tired, my sleep is restless, limbs a bit jerky and I'm waking early 7am.Yawning a lot. D2

16.     Waking up earlier despite dark mornings. Feeling very awake on opening eyes, somehow more awake. D2

8.      Fitful sleep, last night. Woke well before dawn, right shoulder and neck painful. D3

10.     Restless sleep, keep waking up. D3

10.     Woke up with hands driving me mad. D3

5.      Woke up at 2am. with constricting pains in abdomen, didn't sleep much. D3

Gen.

[4,8,7,   Waking up feeling tired. D4

13,15,? ]

10.     Woke up about 4 times during the night, scratching my hands. The itching gets worse with the heat of the bed. D4

8.      Waking up with itchy toes. D5

10.     Restless sleep, tossing and turning, physically uncomfortable. Going to sleep fine, but wake up and toss and turn. Feel like I'm waking every 5 minutes all night long. D5

8.      At night I'm wide-awake, restless. Mind still going, busy, busy. Don't feel like I've had a long, deep sleep. D7

17. Disturbed restless sleep. Mind busy. Tossing and turning in bed, legs fidgety. I'm hot and feel cold, so I pull covers up around my head and then feel too hot. Don't feel as if I've had a long, deep sleep.  D7

17. Waking up in pain, around 3am. Can find no comfortable, pain free position, worse lying on right side. Knee to chest position agg. pain in my abdomen.  D15

10. Good night's sleep, but woke feeling tired.  D10

11. Unrefreshing sleep.  00

Gen.

[7,8,17, Having late nights, staying up reading until the early hours.
10.]  D15

4. Overwhelmed by sleep; need to lie down immediately.  D17

Kept waking last night with aching right shoulder / arm. Couldn't turn my head it was so stiff. Agg. by confrontation with boyfriend, in which I became very emotional.  D17

8. I lay in bed unable to sleep last night. My chest, my breathing all felt odd, irregular. I kept getting palpitations. Perhaps I'm anaemic.  D20

8. Going to bed really late. Not sleeping well, only managing a few hrs. Either, not managing to go to sleep or waking in pain.  00

11. I'm so tired, come home from work, sit down and go to sleep. It's like Knackerlepsy.  M2

10. Snoring in evening, after falling asleep in my armchair.  00

7. Can't stay awake I'm so tired. Yawning a lot.  M2

13. Woke in the night thinking I'm going to die.  M2

8. I keep falling asleep ever time I sit down. It was a heavy sleep that kind of dragged me in to it.  M2

8. Not sleeping well due to cold weather.  M2

2. Feel deathly tired. I just have to sleep. But wake up next morning feeling as if I haven't slept properly, still feeling so tired. 00

8. I hardly slept with the pain {left thigh}. I couldn't find a comfortable position. The night seemed so long and miserable. M2

7. Not sleeping very well, even when I'm, knackered I can't fall asleep Keep waking up. M2

8. I was burning hot but any slight movement of covers seemed to threaten the supply of heat and made me shiver. I slept fitfully; strange images filled my head. M2

7. Woke up at 6.30am, couldn't stop coughing, or go back to sleep. M3

4. Couldn't keep my eyes open. Fell asleep while typing poems. M3

4. Start to fall asleep at 10pm. Can't stay awake. M3

7. Can't sleep due to itch of thrush, one hour on then wake up. Have another hour, and then wake up all night. I'm so tired. M4

17. Restless sleep. Waking up through the night. Wake up sweating, dripping with sweat, worse lying on front. M4

4. When I have to sleep, I HAVE to sleep. Real exhaustion. M4

15,17. Can't sleep on my back. 00

8,17. Can't sleep, too much nervous energy. M4

2. Sleep is deep, but wake up feeling worse than when I went to sleep. 00

4. Wake up in the early hrs. With a feeling of discomfort, I can't pin down; then I can't sleep. M4

7. Woke up thinking I feel dehydrated, with no reason. Pounding headache and raging temp. M7

8. Waking up wanting to go to the toilet. 00

# Dreams

<u>Week before proving.</u>

8.    Dreamt of a large tidal wave coming. I was with a friend, an older lady who is very sensible and down to earth. We were watching for specific signs of the Great incoming tide, so we could take appropriate action. We were responsible for the safety of others.

8.    I was in Canada with my ex-husband's family, travelling in a car or train. There was loads of water outside like a river and it was swelling up. It kept pouring into the open window over me. The water was strange, thick, oily, glutinous and shimmering.

8.    I was crossing a big busy road in London, a crossroads near to where I grew up. It was night. Someone stopped and asked the way to Sunnyside School, where my mum used to attend. I didn't know how to get there. We were standing in the middle of the road, so I suggested we look in a phone book. She didn't want to. Suddenly I thought it's not my problem, it's hers to solve.

16.    Lots of dreams but they are slipping almost as soon as I open my eyes.

1.    Dreamt of the death tunnel and woke in the morning feeling that I'd accepted my death.

9.    Busy dreams.   D2

16.    1. A calf was frightened and was missing its mother. I could tell what it felt by looking at it, no words, just communion.

2. Going to the loo, flushing out the body's physical and emotional shit. D2

10.    I was late for work. Busy dream, lots of visitors.   D2

8.  I was walking down my road, then the scene changed and I was charging down some steps, then into narrow streets. Scene changed again, more streets. I knew I could change it, my dreams and my life.  D2

17. Saw a rainbow arched over the world and watched as it continued under the earth, to form a mirror of above.  D2

10. I found hidden treasure underground. The opening to the underground chamber was in a churchyard, amongst the gravestones. I had the feeling this treasure was either hidden or found during WW II but it was ancient treasure.  D3

8.  I was standing in the middle of a road where three streets meet, close to where I used to live.  D3

8.  I was driving through streets in N, Ireland, close to where my ex- husband grew up. The roads were deserted as I drove on main roads, country roads, crossing through villages and towns and near the border. Later I had to drive back. I got confused and thought I was lost.  D3

16. Strong dreams, like a real other life, but not graspable. But a sense of their deep meaning and significance. Much more "real".  D4

1.  A man in my window kept changing from a little man to an owl. I was laughing at him, taking the Mick. He said, "something is going to happen to you." He was very menacing.  D5

8.  I was in a house with a family and water was soaking through the upstairs ceiling, great damp patches were appearing. A decision was made that it was time to move elsewhere.  D6

8.  We went to visit a couple. A large gathering of like-minded people. Their house revolved, on a turntable base, a large bungalow with many large windows. It spun around, not on a fixed axis, but glided all over the plot. It was as if it was attached to a moving arm. The couple spoke of moving.  D6

8.     Woke in the middle of the night with:
I was on a small motorbike, about to come out of a small entrance at the foot of the hill, turning left. It was dark and my headlamp was lit. I noticed headlights of a car approaching over the brow of the hill. I decided I could make it, put my foot down and there was no power at all, although my headlight still shone. I pulled back into a garage through wooden doors. I closed them and became aware of my partner behind me, touching me. Suddenly a large spider stepped on to my chest and ran across me sideways. I started shouting and woke myself up with "I'm going mad!" and I was facing the opposite direction.   D7

7.     ...of a dog.

10.     Caught a coach to somewhere. Spent a day at my destination. Time to go home, coach had gone. There was a space on a second coach, not going straight home but in the general direction.   D10

5.     Tidal wave, everyone screaming. I rode through it. I saw it coming behind me and I was quite happy. I held my breath and came up, down again and up three times. Didn't think I was going to die. If I die it's not so bad.   D12

17.     Regret over not spending enough time with my children.   D12

17.     Away from home, I'd lost my suitcase in which were all my clothes and belongings. However, my jewellery came back to me.   D14

17.     My son dreamt his legs were paralysed.   D15

12.     Threw my angel picture in the bin. I got really annoyed and then woke up, but the dream carried on.   D24

8.      With my two sons [as children] and pushing ex-husband in his wheelchair. We were in a port. The roads were dry, white and stony. As we rounded a bend, saw a huge body of water coming towards us. It was travelling very fast and I was concerned about getting the children and ex. safely out of the way. I didn't panic. I had to do my best, but if the wave caught us it was fate / destiny and out of my hands.   D26

12.     Saw my Dad [deceased] we were v. close. The sea was extremely full and we were standing at the edge. It mountained up and became a tidal wave. The sea went white, slightly foamy [like detergent effluent]. It was warm, safe, like walking through mist.   M2

8.      I was in front of my Grandfather's house [long deceased], packing, as we were moving. We put a big bag of rubbish out, there was a bit of a panic as we weren't certain where to put it. It had to be in the right place otherwise the dustman wouldn't take it. I was waiting for my Uncle, when a white Mini arrived, was this him? A young man dressed in white overalls and a white cap walked past, carrying a pot of white paint, a roller and a paint brush.   M2

17.     I fell into the primordial ocean, it felt warm and safe.   M2

9.      Dreamt of owls, it felt symbolic.   M2

8.      With my son and grandson, we were climbing into a house. The construction was strange and so was the perspective. Beams, steeply sloping floors and holes in the ceilings. We met a women sitting at a computer, who told us that she was recreating an experience she'd had. She said she'd been wearing her "Dress?" a pale pink, skin tight designer dress with flowers on the hem, and had fallen down a chute. She said it was like a birthing experience and was in raptures over it.   M2

8.      I was living in a small cottage that had grounds large enough for a large manor house.   M2

8. Saw a wonderfully light flaky pastry filled with confectioner's custard. I had no desire to eat it. M2

8. Saw myself and my two sons on a beach looking at the remains of a body, it was emaciated and had been dead awhile. We all knew it was my ex-husband and it felt like an action replay. All washed up. M2

8. I was standing in the centre of a football stadium with someone. They pointed to a row of seats and told me this was where a fire had started, which then spread to the centre of the stadium. M2

8. I go to use a very public toilet. Other women are hassling me, peeing over the short door. I tell them to go away. To my surprise I'm menstruating [it's been 7-8 months since I've had a period]. I sit on the loo, only to find I've peed down the back, outside the pan. When I look I see its blood. My cat appears, rubs against me and the toilet. The right side of her face nuzzles the puddle area, but when she walks away instead of red blood on her face, I see it is blue. M2

8. ...chatting with a friend whose just had twins. They're lying on the ground in the street. One of the twins begins to roll down a pebbly slope and I rescue it. I offer to help by carrying one of the twins, as my friend has to get home. I pick one up, it's a girl. As I walk the baby gets heavier and heavier and I begin to regret helping. It is a much longer journey than I first thought. When I look the baby is the size of a 5-6 yr. old. M2

8. I'm in L.A. on a beach. It's a strange set up, there are high sand walls around which gives everyone a compartment to sit in. Everyone is friendly and there are many film stars around. It is almost time to catch a plane home, but first I want to visit a desk to apply to adopt a child. I'm first in line, but don't have the correct documentation. I find my driving license, try to hand it over, but she's dealing with someone else now. I get angry and shout, " If my papers aren't good enough, I won't take a baby. Fuck you." I storm off. My friend in a non-

emotional way calms me down and I try again, her the diplomat by my side. The woman stamps my papers and shows me a picture of the baby. I'm horrified the photo is of an old handicapped women. She has permed fair hair and looks pathetic. I have a mental picture of me dragging her around by her right arm until she dies, having to feed her and toilet her. This doesn't carry the joy of a new baby and I'm not sure whether I want the responsibility.   M2

17.   Recurring, of being disembowelled. Or pierced by a sword / spear in my liver or through right lower rib cage to heart.   M3

17.   Driving home in the dark, I notice a white stone at the side of the road. Stop car and go over to it. I notice a small hole in the ground in front of the stone and thrust a smooth stick / rod into the hole. The road is so familiar but I hadn't ever noticed this large white standing stone before.   M3

10.   We were in India and there was a swarm of wasps. We were trying to peg down a tent, but I realised they'd come under it. I looked across and saw this palace. There were lots of people mulling about. I decided to go over to the palace and stay there until the swarm had gone.

Looking out the windows everyone was getting stung. But there was no panic. Yet, if I have a fear it is of wasps!   M3

17.   My car was stolen while I was away lecturing. I'd left the car whilst finding directions, and had left everything in it except my shoulder bag. Decided to walk to my destination. Man on bike told me that there is a station up there. He came with me and I gave him my bag to look after while I bought a ticket. When I returned both he and the train had gone.   M3

8.   Visiting North Pole / Arctic Circle to make a presentation at a conference. I was very well dressed. My ex-boyfriend was there with his wife. Couldn't get to talk to him, he had become so dependant on her (opp. of real life), crippled with arthritis.   M4

4.   Lot's of baby dreams. In some I'm pregnant.   M4

8.      …of being pregnant.   M4

17,7.   I was pregnant, felt really nice.   M4

17.     I was to divorce my husband.   M4

17.     In an alien landscape, strange vegetation. I fall into a bog, almost impossible to pull myself out. I'm going to sink under the mud. I grab at the vegetation, which is like plaited rope. But do not have the energy to pull myself out.   M4

17.     Driving along the coast with my sister-in-law. Want to stop and have a swim, it's such a beautiful day, blue sea and sky. Have to drive back the way we came to find a spot. Finally succeed but now we are in the mist. Swim through the mist and someone comes to me and cuddles me, doesn't feel human, yet extremely loving, affectionate, caring towards me. Swim into a building, custom built for 'handicapped' mentally and physically.   M4

8.      I was at a very busy gathering. Our group was gathered in a circle and prover 11 was giving each of us a gift, a symbol in 3D.   M4

17.     …of pyramids{Egyptian},outside looking at one, now inside one.   M4

8.      Remembered my friends' ancient names. A glimpse of us all from an ancient time.   M4

17.     Falling into a black hole, a feeling of infinite nothing. Found it terrifying at first. I looked for the earth, but saw only emptiness where she had once been. I felt a cry of despair and woke.   M4

4.      I was at the theatre; Sarah opened the doors and said to the waiting audience, "I hope you know what this show is, because I haven't a clue." Very unlike her. She was decorating the flat at the theatre, painting poetry on the wall.   M5

4.      I was in a dodgy area and it was getting dark, but trying not to worry. Enormous gusts of wind blew me off my feet. I kept flying away. I called to a man in a suit to hold on to me, feeling awkward because he was a stranger. He was willing to help. Another gust of wind and along came someone I knew from the theatre. He rescued me. He felt like an old friend, he stood behind me and hugged me. We laughed. I realised that I felt easy, comfortable and joyful with him, in a way I haven't been in years. M5

4.      I had this baby that I forgot I had. Whilst changing it's nappy, noticed Jules presiding over this like a man of wisdom / position. He put his hand in the nappy / shit, like a blessing. I said, "It's only my milk." M5

17.     I was in a bar/restaurant with a nice friendly group of women. Next in car with my partner, I'm in the passenger seat. I notice Harrison Ford! who I knew was recovering from a bad accident. He was looking good and I pointed him out to my partner. He was with his wife who had her face covered by a hat. Suddenly he looked down into the car at me, our eyes locked and we connected.

Back in the bar, sitting eating with my new friends, he comes and sits next to me and kisses me passionately. Over the next few moments thousand of years of communication pass between us, all without words. He disappears. Next day in the foyer there is a letter for me. I'm aware of my partner hanging around, knowing something is going on. I manage to disappear to read the letter in private. It began, "I have to be with Pia (wife) because she is my mother, but I love you, always have and always will." The letter became lots of little metal (gold/ silver) figures and symbols attached to the paper. At the bottom two rings, our wedding rings and angels, "You are my angel. I love you forever".

Next we are hiding in a toilet/shower cubicle. I say, "I must talk to you before you leave". I tell him it is time to grow up and leave mother, to reunite with anima and become whole. He pulls me towards him and we melt into each other, twins reunited! M10

2.	Disturbing dreams, unrecalled, except one in which I had a tumour on my chest, level of the thymus gland (? immune system) 00

2.	Lots of vivid dreams. 00

10.	Vivid dreams. 00

17.	Active dreams, significant to the present situation. 00

10,8.	Dreaming lots. 00

17.	Voice in dream saying, " We can never die." 00

17.	Of eyes, sometimes Egyptian-eye of Horus, two almond eyes looking at me. 00

17.	Feeling loved and cared for, safe. A feeling of immortality. 00

17.	Images of torture, people, including me, being disembowelled, burnt at the stake. It feels like past life stuff, as if we are being persecuted for our knowledge. Like Galiano Bruno, Jeanne d'Arc...et al. 00

1.	I was with a young girl who was so frightened because she had a spider on the inside of her muslin, flowing, white dress. It looked like a black widow spider. I was trying to calm her so that I could release the spider, without harming it. I was not afraid. 00

1.	I was at school and there were four young lions. One was black. People were trying to catch them and put them in a safe place. I was observing. I was told to stand on a high wall but I said it was not a safe place. I felt no fear because they were not aggressive. I was fascinated at the clarity of this vision. 00

# Fever

| | |
|---|---|
| 17,10. | Chilly shivering up back.  D1 |
| 2. | Shivery down back of neck and spine.  00 |
| 8. | Feel cold one moment and hot the next.  D2 |
| 5,10. | Feeling hot and cold.  D11 |
| 8. | Burning hot in bed, yet any movement of the covers and I was shivering. At 2am I took my temp, it was 100 F.  M2 |
| 17. | Feel feverish, hot but occasionally very cold, agg. by and very sensitive to drafts.  M2 |
| 8. | Woke up feeling nauseous, with a raging temp.  M2 |
| 15. | Feel feverish, first hot then cold.  00 |
| 4. | Felt generally feverish.  M4 |
| 7. | Raging temp. Felt hot and cold.  M7 |

# Perspiration

| | |
|---|---|
| 5. | Having hot sweats.  D1 |
| 4. | Have been very sweaty, smelly.  D17 |
| 17. | More sweaty than normal, slightly smelly, particularly under arms. Smells sweet, musky or putrid, sour. Worse after exertion, mental or physical.  M2 |
| 17. | Feet have been sweaty, smelly (cheesy).  00 |
| 17. | Night sweats, dripping with sweat, worse lying on front.  M4 |

# Skin

**Gen.**

[7,8,5,10, 1,17,14] General itchiness felt all over the body, or wandering over various parts. D1

11,2. Spots and boils on skin in general, not coming to anything. 00

4. Prickling / itching in my legs and over ribs, felt like shingles. D1

4. Hands covered with contact dermatitis after cutting trees and getting scratched. Itchy and spotty. D2

4. Hands really itchy and red. Woke up with them driving me mad. D3

4. Itching gets really bad with heat. Not bad during the day, but in evening becomes itchy. D4

8. Toes of both feet itchy on waking. Rash, lumpy, hot red dots under the skin. D6

7. Incredible itch, even voluptuous around area where I'd had a boil, left upper arm - vaccine site? D7

7. Bitten by a nit, got inside my dress and bit all over my back. Red raised lumps, very itchy and sore. D12

17. Had a day of jaundice, skin turned yellow, as did urine. D16

8. Incredibly itchy arms on and off for approx. last two days. D28

14. Slightly itchy feeling under surface of skin. M1

8. Boil on solar plexus. Don't feel it will come to anything. M1

7. Have shingles, lower rib cage left, spreading to navel and then right side. Blisters burst, discharge oozes and becomes crusty; sometimes bleed a bit. Blisters burst and spread. It's agg. by touch, I can't wear any clothes next to it. M2

7. Boils on bum that don't come to anything. Red, raised, hard and sore, but blind. M2

17. Skin around waist felt as if I had shingles, a sore, prickly sensitivity; agg. any clothes around my waist. Lying on my back agg. it. M2

16. Eczema type rash on inner thighs, red and itchy, slightly raised. M2

7. There is scabies raging through my village. Both my son and ex-husband have it. Itching all over the body, wherever there is hair; a maddening itch. M2

1. Feels lumpy under my skin. M3

17. Granular feeling under skin, in particular over upper chest. Eruption red, raised and inflamed in middle of sternum. Which reminds me of an experience I had as a child, swimming in the sea. People began to leave the water scratching all over. I soon realised why, it was as if I was being bitten by minuscule bugs all over my body. I suffered an irritating rash all over my body for months, that no doctor could diagnose. A year later I was left with a slight itchy rash / sensitivity on upper chest, just like the one I have now.

The incident was brought up over dinner last night and my friend, who is a journalist, told of the leaks of nerve gas from a military installation, just around the corner from where I'd been swimming, many of which he'd reported. He wondered whether I'd been contaminated by mustard gas or sarin. M3

2. Have been getting patches of ringworm, on face and various parts of body. Very itchy. M4

7. Boil on left calf didn't come to anything. Sore, red and hard, 1 inch in diameter. M4

17. Patch of ringworm left side leg, level with knee. Very itchy, raised, red. Worse for heat and scratching. M5

17. Skin looks yellow / sallow, particularly right hand and lower arm. M5

8,17,7. Getting boils, red, hard and painful, not developing, throughout the proving.

# Generalities

8.    Feel very warm. Glowing with warmth, which seems to be coming from inside. 1$^{st}$. $^1/_2$ hr.

17.   Increase in body temp. 1$^{st}$. $^1/_2$ hr.

7.    Feel cold.   D1

17.   Feeling chilly.   00

12.   Feel warm.   D2

8.    Experience sudden waves of heat on and off throughout the day, not hot flushes. I often feel cold, and then within $^1/_2$ hr. feel very flushed.   D6

8.    I was burning hot in bed yet any slight movement of the covers seemed to threaten the supply of heat and made me shiver. A furnace burned inside me. All day I had been hot and thirsty for water. Despite the heat I wanted to wrap up warm, but my head had to be clear of the covers.   M2

17.   Not feeling the cold, due to inner feeling of warmth.   M3

12.   I haven't been cold all winter; it's been so unnaturally warm.   M4

17.   Feel I've lost weight.   D3

8,1.  Have lost weight.   00

7.    Seem to be losing weight.   D12

16.   More thirsty than usual. Need for water and recognition of that need. Not very hungry for breakfast.   D1

16.   Needed a chocolate fix this evening. Very rare.   D2

17.   Off citric foods.   D3

17.   More hungry than normal.   D3

8.    Off greasy foods. Can even smell the fat in cheese. Sweet and fatty foods leave a taste in my mouth. Unfresh stale taste.   D3

17.   Off greasy / fatty foods.   D3

1.      I can't eat fats.   00

5.      Didn't eat much all day and minimal fluid intake.   D3

5.      Drinking plenty of water.   D5

8.      No desire for chocolate or any sweet things.   D5

10,17.  Desire choc.   D7

8.      Thinking I'm going to eat healthily but eating crap.   D7

17,2.   Off alcohol.   00

7,2.    Off coffee.   00 { Note coffee agg. when used as an antidote.}

12.     Desire crisps.   M1

17.     Agg. fats, pasties, anything with butter in it.   M1

11.     Haven't enjoyed the excessive foods and drink of Christmas, normally I love the indulgence.   M2

17.     All foods seem to agg. abdominal symptoms but especially root vegies, vegie stew.   M2

17.     Little appetite / interest for food.   M2

17.     Off spicy things.   M2

17.     Desire for crisps.   M2

17.     Feel like I'm not digesting food properly.   M2

11.     Haven't wanted to drink alcohol. Have been worrying that I may be addicted.   M2

7.      Don't want to drink alcohol.   M2

11.     Have desired and have been drinking lots of water.   M2

8.      I was very dry so I drank copious amounts of water and was still thirsty.   M2

17.     Burning thirst.   M2

17.     Have been cutting down on stimulants. Wanting to clear my body of toxins, in the hope of regaining some kind of energy level. But also worrying that I might have become addicted, especially to smoking and tea.   M2

7.     Have stopped smoking and cut out tea. Not a conscious decision.  M3

2.     Feel like I do when I'm pregnant, off anything that is bad for me.  M3

13.    Have been very, very thirsty for water. Come home from school and drink a pint of water and I'm still thirsty.  M4

7.     Have been eating sugar / chocolaty things and attracted to whisky and alcohol in general.  M4

2.     I'm drinking more alcohol than normal. Frequently $^{1}/_{2}$ a bottle of red wine a night. Feeling better for it.  00

8.     Food is weighing heavy on me. I haven't been hungry at all. M4

9.     Didn't eat much during this proving, a real change.  00

7.     Off grapes.  M4

1.     Sorting out my diet, have cut out butter and sugar.  M4

7.     My tolerance for any stimulants has been lowered, in particular alcohol.

       I can't stand the smell of coffee, alcohol or tobacco smoke. I'm very sensitive to smells now.  M7

17.    I'm eating well, but seem unable to put on weight. Feel thin, fragile, as if food not nourishing me.  M5

17.    Feeling dehydrated, much better after drinking water. Felt rehydrated, skin looked as if re-hydrated.  M3

8.     I feel dehydrated, as if my brain is shrinking, drawing away from inside my skull.  M4

7,17.  Taking more showers and feeling invigorated after.  M4

2.     From the moment the remedy arrived, I felt lousy. I felt tired all the time.

12.    Extremely tired, yet restless. Jerky limbs.  D2

8.     Quite a physical day, sorting and shifting stock. Felt good physically.  D2

5.     Very energetic day physically.    D3

9.     Feel tired, drained.    D3

12.     Limbs feel stiff and tired.    D3

8.     Feel very tired. Legs aching, knees and soles of feet.    D5

4.     I've had a very physical week, riding 3 times, singing,dance class, felt good about being so physical.    D7

12.     Tendency for my bones to ache, better for a hot bath.    D7

1.     Have flu, had to go to bed, ache all over.    D11

17.     I just had to sit down due to an overwhelming feeling of tiredness. Yet my mind still active, planning, organising. Very tired, yet driven.    D14

8.     Feeling tired, drained of energy, last few days.    D17

17.     I'm exhausted and with it suffering aches in my bones, my back, my shins, ankles, feet and hands. It's a dragging ache. D24

2.     I went out for supper and took fruit juice as I was driving. Next morning woke feeling dreadful. Partner said I looked like I had a bad hangover. I felt exhausted, had an headache and my bones ached. It got worse and worse as the day went on.    00

2.     Constant feeling of having a hangover. Wake up feeling tired and listless.    00

2.     Slow to get going in the mornings.    M2

17.     Feeling generally sluggish.    M2

2,17.     I feel toxic.    00

11.     I'm so tired, come home from work, sit down and go to sleep. It's like Knackerlepsy.    M2

7.     My energy is sluggish, I feel heavy, dragging myself around. M2

11.     Have had more colds / flu bugs over last two months, than is normal for me.    M2

11. Flu like aches in joints and neck.  M3

15. Flu hadn't completely gone before it returned. Exhaustion, fever, chest infection.  M3

8. Fleeting pain like strain / sprain, from shoulders to arms and then all through the rest of my body, ending in my toes.  M3

5. I've been predominantly full on, and then I get very tired. Feeling extremes of energy, all or nothing.  M3

7. Almost impossible to keep awake all day. I have to lie down.  M3

17. Have felt an increase in nervous energy.  M3

17. Feel like I'm suffering from nervous exhaustion.  M3

9. Feel physically relaxed {not the usual const. body tension}.  00

12. I have boundless energy.  M4

8. Keep wanting to sit down and going to sleep.  M4

15. Sometimes I feel so weak I think I'm going to collapse.  00

5. I'm completely exhausted, working like a dog, really busy, plus children and husband not here to help.  00

4. When I have to sleep I <u>have</u> to sleep, real exhaustion. This alternates with periods of frantic activity.  M4

13. Suffering chronic tiredness.  M4

2. I feel deathly tired, really wiped out.  00

17. I'm chronically tired. I feel I'll never have any energy again. I'm totally depleted.  M4

2. My daughter is suffering extreme exhaustion, has swollen glands - neck, under arms and in groin, and has a constant dull headache. She looks ghostly pale / sallow. It looks like glandular fever.  00

17. Gen. feeling of stiffness throughout body, pelvic bone aches and feels stiff.  M4

4. I'm suffering chronic stiffness, even dancing, which I love, seems too robust. M4

8. I long for fresh air, but it's still raining. I keep standing by the open door gulping lung fulls of air. M2

2. I've noticed I feel fine when the sun is shining, but a few days of grey skies and all the symptoms begin again. 00

17. Since the sun as been shining I've felt great, very optimistic, getting back to normal. M4

17. It's rained and rained and it's really getting me down. Even physical symptoms are returning. M6

17. I'm having recurrent feeling of being blocked on all levels. I resolve problems, but I don't move on. Stomach feels blocked, bloated. Nose is blocked with catarrh… M7

2. All my glands feel watery. 00

Gen. Extreme tiredness, exhaustion.

8,7,17. Agg. by chemicals.

Gen. Extremes of energy, frantic activity alternating with absolute exhaustion.

Gen. Itch, general feeling of itchiness.

Gen. Restlessness day and night.

Gen. Feel as if coming down with flu.

Gen. Muscular ache , whole body.

Gen. Provers having symptoms that don't develop. Boils / styes that don't come to a head. Muscular twinges, aches, slight headache as if getting a cold, but nothing develops. As if immune response too weak to throw up symptoms.

Gen. Recurrence of proving symptoms, month three.

8. Just as I thought the proving was over, it all started up again. M3

Gen. Thirsty.

Gen.    Desire water.

<u>Acute- Vignette of spectrum.</u>

7.    It happened so suddenly. Woke up thinking I feel dehydrated
{no reason}. With a pounding headache and raging fever.
Couldn't shift it for 28 hrs. At first I had a pain in chest, heart
level. If I moved or walked it was very painful, incredibly
tender. I panicked, thought I had lung cancer. Then it moved
down to my stomach / solar plexus and then to my abdomen.
Felt slight nausea. I was really ill. Drank loads of water. A
week later I got shingles again, less severe, only a patch, more
of an itch than painful. Two weeks later got a cold, chest
infection, coughing up green sputum. Throughout, felt very
tired, exhausted.    M7

# Meditations

16. Found meditation quite hard as I just keep drifting into images and thought patterns. D3

12. During meditation I thought what if the great pyramid is not just a pyramid but extends into the ground in a mirror image to form a diamond shape. Maybe the internal below structures mirror the above ones. D2

1. Whilst quietly meditating a large black cat came and sat at my feet. This felt like an extremely powerful ally. M1

10. Saw three red beaded knuckles coming for me. {This was before the friction burn on my knuckles.} M3

17. I was in the dark - saw an open door ahead of me and through it a beautiful verdant land. I wanted to be there but realised that I was not going to be allowed. At this point I was shot through the forehead. M5

17. ...found myself in a hall, a library, it had a wispy feel...walls painted powder blue. It was a very comfortable place to be. I didn't want to read so I meditated. I saw a lotus blossom unfolding in front of me. Above it a figure with wings outstretched, at first golden then the wings became spectral, layers and layers of colour. His/her gown at the hem began to form a sphere, which dropped from the gown like an egg; it was earth, then another and another planet.

    I felt wings growing on my back and also became a rainbow-winged creature. I looked down at myself shimmering in a vast indigo space, layers and layers of colour like veils or shafts of light dancing in space

    ...back down by a river where I was taken across in a boat. The boatman was a tall, exquisitely beautiful man, robed in a dark green velvet cloak. 00

# Anecdotal Information

Night of proving, wild and windy. Very stormy. Taken in a house overlooking a boiling sea.

Day after proving, flash floods in Spain and Portugal.

4.  This poem arrived within days of starting the proving. I don't know why, but I think it is linked.

## Beyond Westminster Bridge

The man in the boiler suit carting bleach
to the top floor washrooms of NatWest Tower
alone saw the rainbow over Chelsea Reach
drift towards Westminster Bridge, as if drawn
to a curve almost as natural as it's own,
then hover and, in the next bright shower,
settle onto the roadway, cutting a swathe
through the morning rush hour, which it bathed

In perfect colours. Alone he rang the Sun
who spiked him as another schizo case
as, on the Bridge, commuters inched ahead, none
sensing the glory about them, or taking delight
even in the unexamined uncut light
which fell on the dull and soulless faces,
glinted on Thames and Embankment, marked
the debris of the City, penetrated the dark

foundations of the City's splendour. Alone
he rang the Commons where a few M.P's
exhausted by overnighting, cursed the phone,
glanced at the bridge, saw nothing save
bleary bands of red and blue-but braved
the air to dance in these to please
the Whips. Alone he sighed, scanned each
miraculous colour one last time, still craved
the prism, turned to his job, applied the bleach.

Colin Archer.   From Renewing the Light.   Peterloo Poets.

99

17.     My 5 yr. old son won 1st prize in a Boots colouring competition, to colour a fiery dragon. Proud mother or what?     D4

        Gold found in big quantities in Devon.     D9

5.      House overrun by mice. Had to kill them with traps. Feel bad about it but resigned.     D5

17.     My husband won the lottery twice [£10 each time!]. He never wins anything, Mr. Pessimism.     D10

        Flash floods in Somalia killing 1,000 people. El Ninho effect blamed.  {El Ninho means Christ child.}     D12

[7,10,8,     There is a noticeable presence of mosquitos and gnats, very
17.]     unusual for this time of year.     D12

12.     The BMA - Cannabis legalised for medicinal use. Brilliant for taking away the pain of labour.     D14

        Boericke "With Cannabis Indica, pain diminishes as if the sound of a bell disappearing into the distance."

        At least 61 western tourists shot dead by machine gun or hacked with knives by fundamentalists in Luxor, Egypt.     D15

        Three weeks into proving and it has rained since taking it.

        Flash floods in Cornwall, 6-8 ft in places.     D25

10.     The electrics went at my husband's college. Blue flashes were seen dancing all around the place.     D25

        Warmest Nov. for 107 yrs.     M1

        Saddam Hussein backs down, allowing weapons inspectors in. But no Americans. Seems to be the end of the current Gulf crisis.     M1

        Meteor lands in Greenland creating a crater a mile wide.     M1

        Newton's rings seen around the moon, seen full moon and day before     M1

8.      My boyfriend's car caught on fire, in the pouring rain.     M1

12.     In Singapore, explosions in the sky like fire bombs. Lightening and thunder together.     M2

100

Son of 7.Despondency-"I'm completely fucked. I've completely fucked my body. I'm depressed. I can't do anything, travel or anything, I'm too fucked. At moment itchy all over due to having scabies" On the edge of anger all the time.   M2

10.     All the symptoms of this remedy have been very intense. Sometimes a speeded up version of bits from all the other remedies we've done [7 separate colours.]   M3

17.     In a conversation about communication technology and computers, idea came that soon we could be fitted with a microphone in our lips that translated everything said, into any language. Also a receptor in our ear, giving us the ability to talk to anyone in the world.   M3

10.     The head was out this week and the kids are running riot, real nasty fights in the playground, kicking doors…Damian the little splodge of poison….[works in a school for learning disabled ] I question whether this is all the result of the vaccines. We've lots of autistic children here who are accepted as being vaccine damaged.   M3

17.     Since taking the remedy have been more aware of the presence of crows and ravens.   M3

12.     Painted my room madder pink [earth red and white emulsion.] M5

12.     I've been drawn to turquoise. My daughter bought herself a turquoise outfit.   M5

2.     I don't want to wear any crystals or use any crystal essences, I haven't for a few weeks. But now I feel the need to wear turquoise, to stop the effects of this remedy. It's the crystal I would use to stimulate the immune system. I remember reading somewhere that turquoise is at the end of its evolutionary cycle and a higher vibration will come in to replace where it left off. Perhaps we still need it to 'hold' the higher vibration into earth? 00

17.     My friend gave me a pair of garnet earrings for my birthday. I haven't taken them off, it feels good wearing them.   00

10.     Wearing garnet earrings. 00

7.     Thought I'd lost the garnet bracelet I'd been wearing, but found it. 00

2.     My son, who has been 'difficult' recently, suddenly became sweet, affectionate, thoughtful after I took the proving. 00

2.     My youngest daughter has just started school. She's gone past tired and is now hyper. I found her building castles at 3 am this morning. 00

8.     House in flames a few doors down from my boyfriend's house. 00

8.     Misty here and rain, rain, rain. Gales tomorrow, serious weather. 00

8.     Caught myself singing "Search for the hero inside yourself,
> Look for the secrets you hide.
> Search for the hero inside yourself
> Then you find the key to your life."
> By M. People.

00

10.     Crises at work, finally all main members of staff called to a meeting, to rectify matters. Told we had to be totally honest yet, soon became apparent that our lips were zipped. I felt such disillusionment; they were accepting bad behaviour from a child who is capable of so much more. The school as gone from something so well run to chaos. 00

2.     I have a spleen imbalance and my solar plexus is way out, normally very strong. 00

16.     Reflexologist has noticed that my solar plexus is well down. 00

9.     Weakness in solar plexus and colon picked up by Reflexologist. 00

4.     Went to Tessa {healer} my solar plexus is weak at the moment. 00

# Accidents

1.	Walked into tree, poked lteft eye with branch. Eye ball swollen.
	D1

5.	My son has a round red patch in his hair about 1 _ inches in diameter, in the centre of his head. His eye is slightly bloodshot. The inner corner is red and shiny like an open wound. Looks like a chemical burn.

	2nd son's knuckle is livid, looks like a burn wound, red and angry. Went pussy and crusty. Led. worked. Lavender soothed.

	All three of my boys seem to be covered in bruises at the moment.	D12

4.	Nearly had an accident, almost fell on top of a car, whilst riding a very dangerous and out-of-control feeling, horse. Was very frightened.	D6

4.	Pulled my back wrestling with a drawer. Then bent over to pick something up and felt the most excruciating pain in lower back right Legs wobbly and keep collapsing. Feel sick. Masseur / Reflexologist tells me it is the muscle in my middle left back that is worse affected and the pain I feel is referred pain.	D9

4.	Son fell off his bike, bad grazes on his hands.	D11

1.	Broke a glass ashtray, very unusual for me to be so clumsy.
	D11

5.	I'm accident-prone at the moment.	D12

7.	Son accident-prone, breaking light switches. Opens doors and the knobs fall off....	D12

10.	Son spilt drink on TV and video and it blew up!	M1

12.	I've been stumbling into things, very clumsy.	M2

10.	Never prone to burns but over last week: 1st, a friction burn left wrist and three knuckles, playing with children at school. 2nd, spat at by boiling fat at school, we were having Chinese. 3rd, I was jolted whilst carrying boiling coffee and teas and spilt them on my arm.	M3

10. Bruises, having been bitten and kicked by children at school. M4

5. My young son has bruises all over at the moment. M4

# Comment from prover No.2

I think this Rx. would be good for those:
- Feeling overwhelmed
- Phobic
- Exhausted, severe e.g. ME
- Nervous exhaustion
- Antisocial, even autistic
- Intolerant, impatient
- Glandular fever

Also for clearing drug overdose/excesses, poisons, toxic food, radiation??
Nervous and immune system problems e.g. MS, Parkinson's disease.
For those severely distressed mentally and emotionally.
- Nervous breakdown
- Paranoia
- Mania
- Depression
- Suicidal tendencies
- Schizophrenia

# Repertory

# Introduction

It is intended that this repertorisation provides a bridge between the proving and the case; an efficient means of accessing salient symptoms and characteristics of this remedy.

The emphasis is on accessibility and clarity rather than to provide an exhaustive account of every detail. We recognise and welcome the need for each homoeopath to add to and interpret these results and to refer to provers symptoms as required.

The repertorisation has been based on Dr. Schroyens 'Synthesis' Edition 7.1. All current rubrics can be found in there, and new rubrics have been included were considered appropriate and necessary. These are highlighted NR and have been evolved to incorporate provers language with the language and style of the repertory, and our sense of the essence of the remedy.

For ease of access I have deliberately presented these rubrics in the bold, italic and plain type style of the repertory to which we have become accustomed. Section headings follow the format of Synthesis 7.1.

At the end of the repertory is a single page theme map, designed to potentise our understanding of the essence of Spectrum.

Further details on methodology can be found in Appendix 5

Dee Lalljee BA Hons (PEAS)
May 2000
Student at The School of Homoeopathy

# MIND

*Acceptance NR*
Ailments from, love; disappointed
Air, mental symptoms amel. in open
*Anger*
Anger, past events, about
Anger, suppressed
Anxiety, business about
Anxiety, future about
**Anxiety, health about**
*Anxiety, hypochondriacal*
Anxiety, morning on waking
*Assertive NR*
Aversion, husband to
Awareness heightened, birds, presence of
Awareness, heightened
Awareness, heightened, animal awareness
Awareness, heightened, of colours NR
*Balanced NR*
**Busy**
Busy, alternating with exhaustion NR
Clairvoyance
Colours, blue, desire for
Colours, blue, desire for, turquoise
Colours, gold, desire for NR
Colours, purple, desire for
Colours, red, desire for
Communicate, inability to
Communication, desire for NR
*Company, aversion to*
Company, aversion to amel. when alone
Concentration difficult
Confidence, want of self
*Confident*
Content
*Creative NR*
*Death, desires*
*Death, presentiment of*
Delusion, angels seeing
Delusion, animals abdomen are in
Delusion, body, dragging down NR
Delusion, body, thin is
Delusion, body, uncomfortable NR
Delusion, born feels as if newly, into the world and was overwhelmed with wonder at the novelty of his surroundings
Delusion, cancer has a

MIND contd.

Delusion, crime, committed a crime, he had
Delusion, desire to rest from the pressures of this world NR
*Delusion, dimension, is in another NR*
*Delusion, disease, that he has an incurable*
Delusion, falling into unconsciousness and death NR
Delusion, fire, house on
Delusion, fire, thinks the world is on
**Delusion, he is separated from the world**
Delusion, hollow, body is hollow, whole
Delusion, intoxicated, he is
Delusion, images phantoms sees, frightful, sleep, while trying to
Delusion, invaded, one's space is being
Delusion, old, aged, feels
Delusion, persecuted, he is
*Delusion, poisoned he has been*
*Delusion, pregnant, that she is*
**Delusion, psychically drained NR**
Delusion, pursued, he was
Delusion, separated body, spirit had separated from
Delusion, small, world felt small under her feet NR
*Delusion, transition, she is in*
Delusion, trapped NR
Delusion, treasure/money, of coming into NR
Delusion, unreal, everything seems unreal
Delusion, vitality, vivid consciousness of usually unnoticed operations, of
Delusions, betrayed that she is
Delusions, criticized she is
*Despair*
**Detached**
Discouraged
Dream, as if in
*Dullness, sluggishness, difficulty of thinking and comprehending*
Estranged; friends and relatives
Euphoria
Exertion; physical, desire
Fear
Fear, burden of becoming a
Fear, cancer of
Fear, death of
Fear, happen something will
Fear, insanity
Forsaken feeling
Home, desire to go
*Hopeful*
*Humility*

MIND contd.
Hurry, haste
*Ideas abundant, clearness of mind*
Ideas, deficiency of
Impatience
**Introspection**
*Intuitive NR*
Irresolution, indecision
Irritability, morning on waking
**Irritable**
Light, desire for,
*Longing, repose and tranquillity, for*
*Memory, weakness of*
*Memory, weakness of, words for*
Mind and body separated
Optimistic
Origins, desire for NR
Overwhelmed NR
Quarrelling, aversion to
Rage, fury
Reading, desires
Rest, desire for
Restlessness, anxious
Restlessness, day
Restlessness, night
*Sadness*
Senses acute
Sensitive, external impressions to all
Sensitive, noise to
*Sensitive, oversensitive*
Spectres, ghosts, spirits, sees
*Storms, excited by NR*
*Suicidal thoughts*
Suicidal thoughts, car, desire to drive into another vehicle NR
Thoughts persistent, night
Tidal wave, sensation of NR
Time, quickly, appears shorter, passes too
Time, timelessness sense of NR
*Toxic  NR*
**Tranquillity**
Truth, desire for NR
Unbalanced NR
Unhurried NR
Unification, sense of unification with universe
Walking, legs feel as though walked for miles NR
Weather, cloudy agg.
*Weeping*

MIND contd.
Weeping amel.
Weeping, desire to

## VERTIGO

**Vertigo**
Morning
*Morning, rising on*
Evening
Walking, while

## HEAD

Brain, aching deep in
*Congestion*
Constriction
Eruptions, margins of hair
Heaviness
Itching
*Pain*
Pain, accompanied by nausea
*Pain, forehead*
Pain, forehead extending to temples
Pain, morning, waking on
Pain, pulsating
Pain, pulsating, forehead
Pain, pulsating, sides, left
Tingling

## EYE

Dryness
Ecchymosis
Heat in
*Heaviness*
*Itching*
Photophobia
Sunken
Sunken, sensation

## VISION

Acute
Colours, bright

## EAR

Itching
Noises in
Noises in, buzzing
Pain
Pain, left

## HEAR

Impaired

## NOSE

*Catarrh*
Catarrh, morning
Coryza, discharge with
Coryza, evening
Coryza, morning
*Discharge, clear*
Discharge, crusts, scabs, inside
Discharge, yellow
Discharge, yellowish-green
Dryness, inside
Itching, inside
**Pain, sore**
Smell, acute
Smell, acute, strong odours
Smell, diminished
Sneezing

## FACE

Discoloration, pale
Discoloration, red
Drawn
Eruptions
Heat, flushes
**Pain, cheek, cheekbones**
Spots
Tension jaw lower

## MOUTH

Dryness
Pain, sore
Taste wanting
Ulcers

# TEETH

Abscess
Breaking off
Grinding
*Grinding, sleep during*
Looseness of
*Sensitive, tender*

# THROAT

Catarrh
**Dryness**
**Pain, sore**
Pain, sore on waking

# EXTERNAL THROAT

Swelling, cervical glands
Thyroid

# STOMACH

Appetite, increased
**Appetite, wanting**
*Distension*
Eructation, ineffectual and incomplete
Gurgling
Hiccough
Indigestion
Nausea
Nausea, eating after
Nausea, morning
Pain, burning
Thirst, burning

# ABDOMEN

Bubbling
*Clothing, sensitive to*
Distension
*Flatulence*
Heat
Pain, cramping
Pain, liver
Pain, pressure agg.
*Pain, stitching*

ABSOMEN Cont.
Pain, stitching, Hypochondria, right
Spleen, complaints of
Swelling, inguinal region
Weakness, sense of

## RECTUM

Boils, anus, near, blind boil NR
Constipation
Constipation, ineffectual urging and straining
*Diarrhoea*
Diarrhoea, involuntary
*Flatus*
Itching
Itching, night
Pain, soreness

## STOOL

*Frequent*
*Thin*
Watery
Yellow

## BLADDER

*Urination, frequent*

## URINE

Colour, yellow, dark
Odour, strong

## KIDNEYS

Pain, aching

## FEMALE GENITALIA

Eruptions, itching
*Itching*
Menses, irregular
*Menses, late*
Pain, uterus
Sexual desire increased

# RESPIRATION

**Breathlessness NR**
Deep
**Difficult**
Difficult walking
Impeded

# COUGH

Morning
Morning, on waking

# EXPECTORATION

Brownish
Greenish
Taste, salty
White
Yellow

# CHEST

Anxiety, in
Burning, chest
Congestion
Eruption, rash, red
Fullness, mammae
Pain
Pain, cramping
Pain, heart, aching
Pain, sides, left
Pain, sore
Pain, sore, bruised, ribs right, last rib under
Pain, sternum
Pain, stitching, heart
Palpitation, heart

# BACK

Coldness, up the back, dorsal region, scapulae between
Cracking, cervical region
*Pain, aching*
Pain, aching, dorsal region, scapulae
Pain, aching, dorsal region, scapulae
Pain, aching, dorsal region, scapulae, extending to shoulders
*Pain, aching, lumbar region*

BACK Cont.
Pain, burning
Pain, burning, cervical region
Pain, cervical extending to shoulders
Pain, cervical region
Pain, cervical, extending to shoulders, right
Pain, dorsal region, scapulae, right, extending to shoulder
*Pain, right NR*
Pain, sore, ribs right, last rib under
Stiffness
Stiffness, cervical region

# EXTREMITIES

Coldness, foot
Coldness, hands
Eruption, hand, pimples itching
Eruption, hand, pimples red
Eruption, thigh, pimples, itching
*Itching*
Itching, foot
Itching, hand
Itching, leg
Itching, upper limbs
Lameness
Pain, aching, hands
*Pain, aching, hips*
**Pain, aching, joints**
Pain, aching, knee
Pain, aching, legs
Pain, aching, lower limbs
Pain, aching, upper arm
Pain, aching, wrists
Pain, dislocated as if, hip, right
Pain, hip, right
Pain, shoulder, left
Pain, shoulder, right
Pain, sore, foot, sole
Pain, stitching, upper arm
Pain, thumb, left
Pimples, itching
Restlessness, leg, accompanied by aching knees NR
Sensitive, lower limbs
Stiffness
Stiffness, fingers
Stiffness, thumb
Swelling, fingers

EXTREMITIES Cont.
Swelling, wrist, nodular swellings
Weakness, hand, left
Weakness, knee, right
Weakness, leg


## SLEEP

*Restless*
Restless, pain with
*Sleepiness, daytime*
Sleepiness, morning
**Sleepiness, overpowering**
Sleeplessness
*Sleeplessness, accompanied by desire to read NR*
**Unrefreshing**
*Waking, early*
Waking, frequent
Waking, heat from
Waking, itching by
Waking, midnight after, 2-3h
Waking, pain with
Waking, thirst by
Waking, urinate with desire to
*Yawning*


## DREAMS

Ancient, of ancient times NR
Angels NR
Animals
Babies, of NR
Busy
Children, about
Clairvoyant
Closet, being on
Crossroads
Dead bodies
Dead relatives
Dogs
Events, past, long
Falling, abyss, into an
Falling, water into
Family, own
Fire
Food
Journey

DREAMS Cont.
Journey, difficulties with
Lions
Many
Moving, of
Owls, of NR
People
*Pregnant, being*
Prophetic
Rainbows
Sea, tidal wave NR
Spiders
Treasure, of finding NR
True, on waking, dreams seem
Unpleasant
Wasps
Water

# CHILL

Chill in general

# FEVER

Morning
*Alternating with chills*
Alternating with chills, night
Fever, heat in general
Motion, amel.
Rest, agg.
Shivering

# PERSPIRATION

Exertion, during
Hot
Odour, sour
Profuse, night

# SKIN

*Discolouration, red, spots*
Discolouration, yellow
*Eruptions, boils, blind NR*
*Eruptions, itching*
Eruptions, ringworm
**Itching**
Sensitiveness

# GENERALS

Activity amel.
Air, open air, desire for
Bathing, amel.
Cold feeling
Dehydrated NR
*Emaciation*
Food & drink, alcohol, desires
Food, agg.
*Food, chocolate, desire*
Food, fat, aversion to
Food, fruit, aversion to sour
Food, spices, aversion to
Food, sweets, aversion
*Food, water, desire*
Hangover, sensation as if from a
Heat, alternating with chills
Heat, flushes of
Heat, sensation of
Heaviness, internally
**Influenza**
Injuries
Irritability, excessive
Jerking, joints in
*Lassitude*
Lassitude chemicals agg. NR
Lassitude, lie down must
Light, amel. Sunlight
*Morning*
*Pain, aching, bones in NR*
Pain, joints of
Pressure, agg.
Restlessness
Rubbing, amel.
Sluggishness, of the body
Strength, sensation of
Tension, internally
Wavelike sensations
**Weakness, enervation**
Weariness
Weather, cloudy weather, agg.
Weather, wet agg.
*Weight, loss NR*

# Theme Map

LIGHT

FIRE

CONNECTED    CREATIVE

ENERGETIC    TRANSFORMATION

| | B A L A N C E D | |
|---|---|---|
| unification | | confident |
| humility | | inspired |
| busy    acceptance | | unhurried   treasure |
| industrious | | journeying |
| vitality | | assimilation |

FOCUS

TRAN-QUILITY   CALM

STRENGTH   BIRTH

TRUTH

| heightened | LIGHT | communication |
|---|---|---|
| awereness | is energy / not substance    enforms / life | origins |
| assertive | | |
| intellect | | introspect |

CLARITY    HOPE

EARTH

**SPECTRUM**
Rainbow Bridge

WATER

TRANSITION          TRANSITION

| | is refracted sunlight    Fire of life | |
|---|---|---|
| poisoned | | invasion |
| criticised | | boundaries |
| the fall | | intuition |

FEAR    LOSS    PAIN

WEAKNESS   DULLNESS

UNDER-FUNCTION

BETRAYAL

| | U N B A L A N C E D | psychically |
|---|---|---|
| death | | drained |
| timelessness | forsaken | overwhelmed |
| different | seperation | irritable |
| dimensions / persecution | | |
| suicide | lack of | |
| incurable | resistance | |

DISORIENTATION

DIFFUSE

DRAINED

DESPAIR    DISCONNECTED

AIR

**DARK**

This is a visual aid to present our interpretation of the themes arising in the remedy Spectrum.

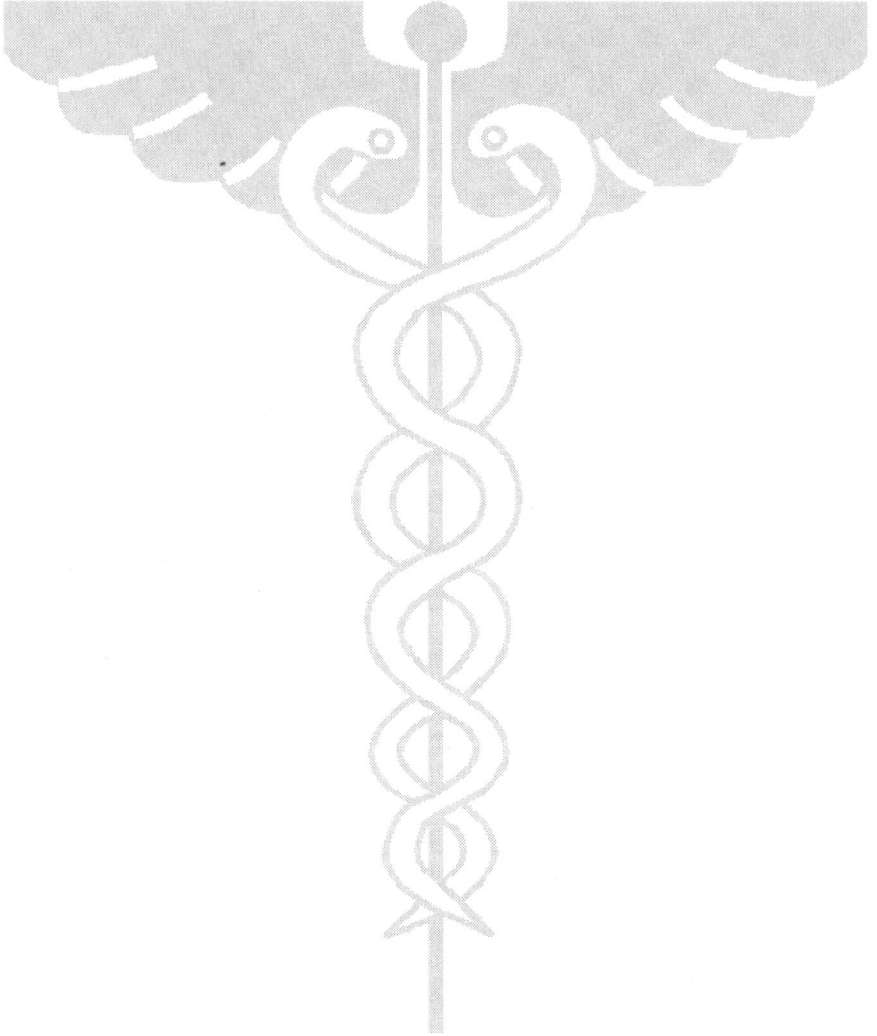

# Notes

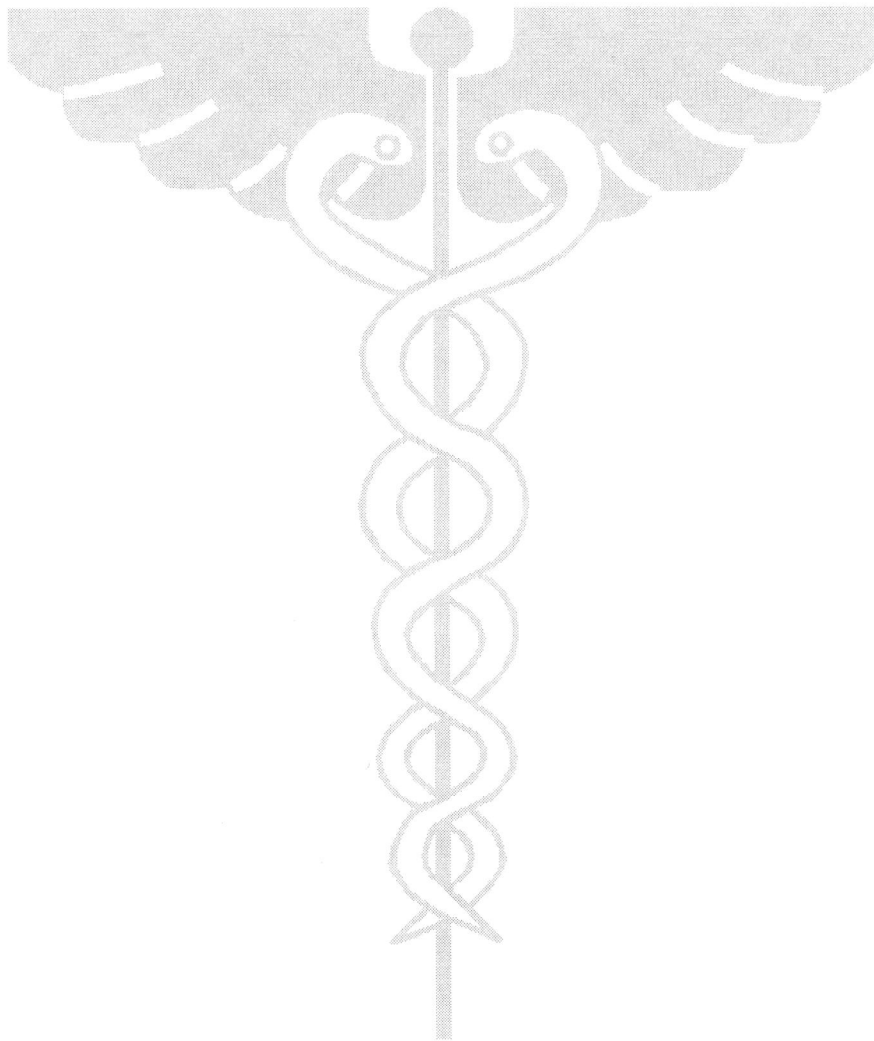

# Notes

# Appendix

# The Astrology of Spectrum

When we first decided to attempt to prove the colours of the visible spectrum, it was suggested that an astrological birth chart be drawn up for each colour as we tested it. Since anything - an idea, a person, a club, a group has a birth (that is, a moment in time when it becomes a physical reality in the manifest world) then it is possible to produce a chart for that 'thing'.

In all, we proved eight remedies - one for each colour and one for the spectrum as a whole - so eight birth-charts were cast. Although each separate proving has its own chart it is worthwhile to consider the very first chart in light of the whole project as it represents the initiatory step in the venture.

One of the most prominent features of that first chart was a conjunction at the IC between the North Node and the planetoid Chiron (pronounced Ky-ron). The IC is the Nadir or lowest point of the chart. As such it represents our roots, home and the soul. By sign and aspect it describes what we are like deep down inside. The North Node indicates purpose and direction and therefore is a symbol of the future. Chiron has been described as the wounded healer. This conjunction, then, implies a healing at a very deep level.

Chiron, in fact, figured quite strongly in most of the charts so I think it important to provide some background information on this planetoid. It was discovered in 1977 and has been called a herald of the New Age. It orbits between Saturn and Uranus. Saturn rules earthy Capricorn and is a great teacher of earthly lessons. It governs time, man-made laws, discipline, establishment and all those solid things that man has manifested here on planet Earth. In effect, Saturn gives us structures by which to live our lives. Uranus, by contrast, enlightens us to possibilities outside of our everyday existence. It shows us different ways of being, shakes us up and is anti-establishment. It usually has the effect of freeing us up in some way. The ruler of Aquarius, and, therefore, the New Age, Uranus is the first of the outer planets that connect us with the collective unconscious. Chiron, then, transiting between Saturn and Uranus can be viewed as the link between these two, very different planets. It links Earth (Saturn) and the heavens (Uranus), or body (Saturn) and spirit (Uranus). Chiron is a symbol for the shaman's rainbow bridge.

In mythology Chiron was a wise centaur and the healer/teacher of Greece's young heroes. He unfortunately became wounded in his leg - the animal part of him that is most connected to the Earth - and despite all his medicinal skills he could not find a cure. Since he was born of the gods, he was immortal and therefore unable to die so suffered great agony and pain. Eventually, Chiron was allowed to change places with Prometheus, which released him to the Underworld.

In Astrology the position of Chiron in one's personal chart gives an indication of where and how one's greatest wound is experienced. Just as importantly, it also reveals the ways in which one's unique skills could be used for the benefit of mankind.

Getting back to the first chart, there is a strong suggestion that this proving venture is concerned with the purpose of healing some very deep wounds. Possibly not only those obtained in early childhood but also those passed on from our ancestors or from previous lives. It also highlights the potential for bringing balance and harmony into play, as the IC, Chiron and the North Node are in the sign of Libra, the Scales.

Moving on to the birth chart of Spectrum (no. 8) the North Node is again conjunct the IC, requiring that we look deep within in order to move forward. Here, though, the conjunction takes place in the sign of Virgo, demanding purification and perfection.

Chiron, this time, is in Scorpio conjunct the Sun. This is real healing of the self! The Sun is the focal point of any birth chart for it is the great light that shines forth and states 'this is me!' and is the energy that establishes one as a separate individual with a power that is unique and special. In this chart the Sun is placed in its own house, the 5$^{th}$, giving it the potential of shining brilliantly with all the playfulness and creativity of a young child. However, in the sign of Scorpio, conjunct Chiron, there is every indication that the real self has been pushed down and buried as a result of a wound that dates back to childhood. There could be some mystery attached to this hurt, perhaps simply because it has been hidden so deeply or maybe because the subject is regarded as taboo. For whatever reason, it lurks in the dark. But here is the opportunity for it to be brought into the light and healed.

There is tremendous power in this configuration. Scorpio has hidden power and the Sun represents the power at the centre of the individual. The sign of Scorpio is noted for its deep reserves of inner strength and the desire to constantly remake itself. Here then, lies the opportunity for total transformation and the square aspect from Jupiter in the 8th house (the natural house of Scorpio) intensifies this. Since the aspect is a square it will require effort, so the healing is not without difficulty. Both Jupiter and Uranus (also in square to the Sun and Chiron) are in Aquarius suggesting that the problems need to be viewed in a totally different way and that perhaps a more objective approach is necessary. Healing of the inner child or deep-seated pain always uncovers powerful emotions. While it is a vital part of the healing process to explore these feelings from the past it is also necessary to understand the hurt from a higher perspective in order to move on. The person who is able to adopt a philosophical attitude or employ a spiritual approach to the subject once the pain has been thoroughly relived has probably more chance of recovery. The placement of Jupiter and Uranus in detached Aquarius affords this potential.

The 8th chart shows most of the planets in one sector of the horoscope, that is, from the 5th through to the 8th house. This area is what astrologer, Howard Sasportas, described as the 'social' part, where 'me in here' meets 'you out there'. This patterning of the chart feels somewhat uncomfortable and rather intense, but also offers hope that 'me in here' can be healed and liberated in order to meet 'you out there' with confidence.

Three of the personal planets, Moon, Venus and Mars are situated in the 6th house. It is here that we examine the practicalities of everyday existence in an attempt to correlate our inner and outer worlds. This is the place where we scrutinise our daily life hoping to create order out of potential chaos. These three personal planets placed here highlight the need to integrate mind, body and feelings in order to operate successfully. Positioned in the sign of Sagittarius, they give an optimistic outlook on everyday life.

Saturn in this chart is the only planet not in the $5^{th}$ - $8^{th}$ house sector. It is found in the $10^{th}$ house in Aries. Although in its own house it is not at ease in Aries. The fire of Aries is somewhat stifled and suggests that the spontaneity and individuality of the self is hampered. However, the discipline of Saturn combined with the initiative of Aries can be very productive in attaining goals. The trine from Saturn to the Moon in the $6^{th}$ confers organisational abilities accompanied by common sense and the sextile to Jupiter in the $8^{th}$ suggests that the opportunity to expand the inner vision and understanding can be promoted in order to enhance belief and confidence in the self.

Pat Neill

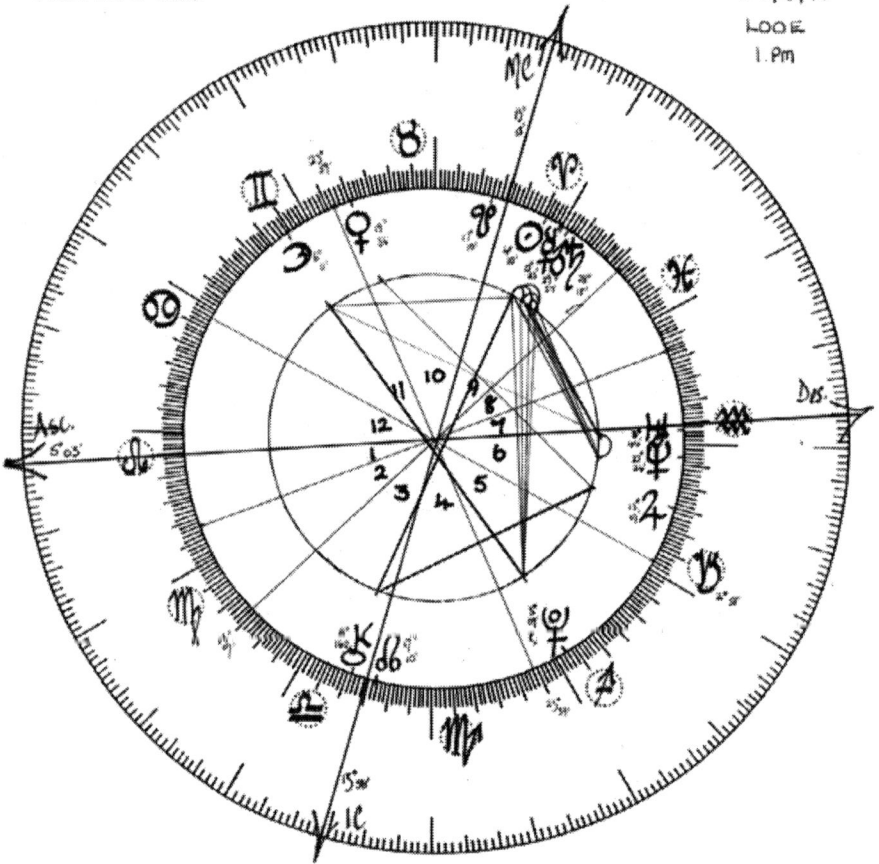

PROVING No.1

24/3/96
LOOE
1.Pm

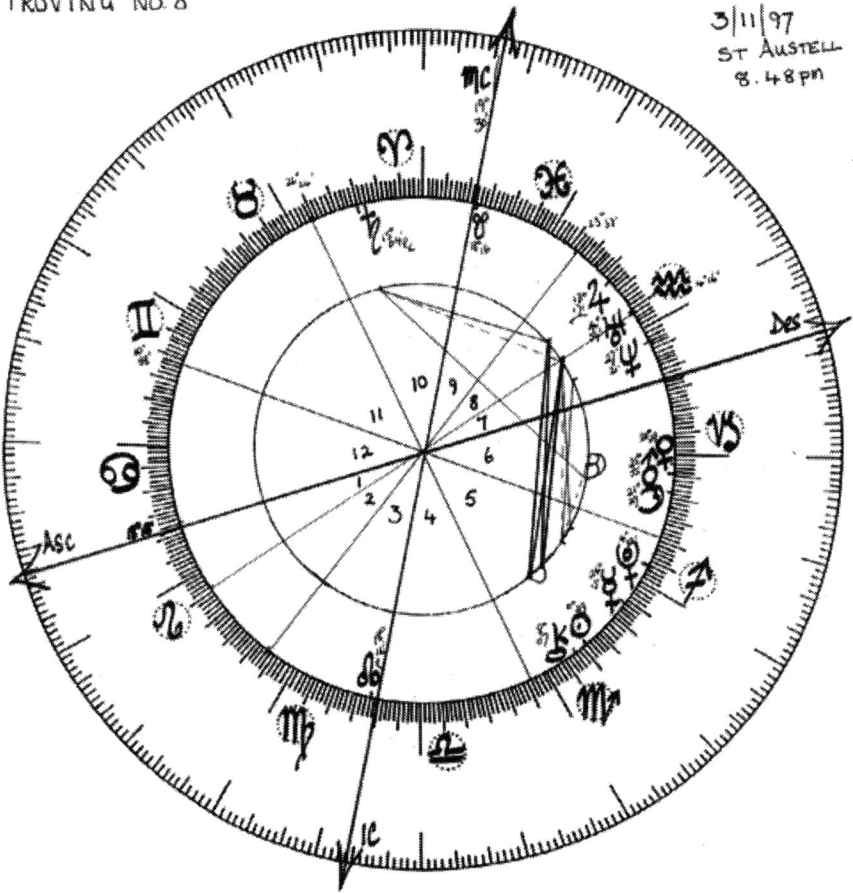

PROVING No. 8

3/11/97
ST AUSTELL
8.48 pm

# The Myth

He was Priest King of the centaurs: a healer, astrologer, oracle and wise teacher of all the young heroes of myth.[1] His name was Chiron, a Master skilled in medicine, music, hunting and warfare. Educated by Apollo, God of the sun and Artemis, Goddess of the moon; he had great wisdom and spirituality.

He taught his noble young acolytes about their personal power through initiation. Only when they had proved their courage by facing their own inner enemies, would they be taught the skills of war. Chiron's pragmatic methods enabled his pupils to win a sense of their personal destiny within the community, thus becoming true leaders and servants of the people. The healer warrior presents a very positive archetype against our present backdrop of savage militarism. *Interestingly a number of provers voiced the need for a new male archetype.*

Chiron founded the Chironium, the ancient healing temple. He was the father of medicine, who taught many, including Aesclepius[2] in the arts of healing. However, one fateful day his friend Hercules paid a surprise visit, having just slain the monstrous Hydra with her nine poisonous heads. Accidentally he grazes the centaur in the thigh with an arrow steeped in the Hydra's blood. The wound is incurable, and so Chiron comes to represent the wounded healer. Through the eye of his wound, his suffering, he can appreciate and understand the pain of others.

As homoeopaths we recognise the similarity to sulphur, the 'medicina' and the 'medicus' who has the illness, is the illness and cures the illness. The Divine Healer {Christ, Chiron, Aesclepius.} who suffers the wound, the persecution, yet also has the potential to heal the universal illness of mankind; the split between above and below[3].

*Suprisingly there is a big psoric quality to this proving. A big itch, boils, scabies,inertia and underfunctioning on all levels. Along with feelings of isolation and separation from the whole.*

1 To the Ancient Greeks he was an Iatromantis.

2 Later Aesclepius was seen as the founder of medicine due to his great skill in surgery and the use of drugs.

3 Ref. Psyche and Substance.

 The Alchemy of Healing.  E.Whitmont.

In another version of the myth Chiron disillusioned by the drunken, unruly behaviour of the other centaurs, poisons himself with one of Hercules' arrows, tipped with a poison he had taught Hercules to make. He returns to his cave in agony unable to die due to his immortality, "poisoned by the collision of his benign nature and the poison of the world."[4]

*Provers felt toxic poisoned by self- inflicted poisons, alcohol, drugs and tobacco and also by environmental pollution. There was also a strong feeling of disillusionment and suicidal thoughts.*

Chiron decides to ask his half brother Zeus if he can exchange destinies with Prometheus who had been chained to the rock of matter, having his liver pecked at by day and healing by night: for stealing the fire of consciousness and sharing it with man. Zeus agrees and knowledge becomes acceptable, no longer a sin.

Meanwhile, Chiron willingly descends into the underworld to face Hades and the lessons of death, transformation and rebirth, sacrificing his life for the greater good of all.

*Some provers felt a fall into the dark night of their soul, to search through their wounds and vulnerabilities. Some saw it as their last task.*

Thanks to Prometheus man was made conscious and thus raised above animals and the rest of creation. However, we have developed our rational {conscious} mind at the expense of our instinctual {unconscious} animal self.

Chiron is one of the many Gods wounded in the leg/thigh or his relationship with physical reality, the leg being that which we must stand on or make our stand in the material world; another, perhaps more familiar, being the Fisher King. We have become separated from the natural world, the very thing that sustains us and gives us life. This schism is creating a wasteland of both our inner and outer environment. Like the centaurs of the myth we are out of control. Our need to manipulate and control the earth, even "torture her secrets from her"{Bacon} has brought us to the brink of annihilation. *The provers dream of an abyss, a black hole where the earth once was, is a profoundly disturbing image, especially if you believe in reincarnation.*

4 Astrology of Fate. Liz Greene.

Despite his immense knowledge and wisdom, Chiron was unable to save himself from the Hydra's poison, because this is the poison of the shadow, which lurks in the deepest recesses of our unconscious mind and contains our deepest wounds-shadows of all the things we have neglected and denied.

Like a true hero Chiron chooses to face the demons of the underworld, in order to learn how to transform the poisons of the shadow and so heal his festering wound. Likewise when we too reach a crisis point, a crossroads in our lives, in order to evolve we need to go not upwards but fall down into the realms of the unconscious, to face the night side of our psyche and our inner monsters.

This is not an intellectual process, for the fear, anger, guilt, grief and so on, have to be experienced, before we can understand and integrate them. Remember Chiron teaches through initiation. What we gain by this process is access to our true potential and a feeling of personal power. Having braved the shadow we find that here also in the unconscious lays the source, that which nurtures our natural abilities and creativity. Not only are our deepest wounds healed, but we are also gifted with the potential to regenerate our lives. We bring the seed of light back from the darkness of the unconscious into the light of consciousness. Chiron becomes the bridge between the two.

One of the aspects of Chiron is of Priest. The ancient word for priest is Pontifex, maker of bridges, the priest being the bridge, mediator between man and his God. However, this priest does not symbolise any orthodox creed. He is a wild creature, half man and half animal, whose temple is a cave in a mountain. "Thus the spiritual law which he transmits is not a collective one distilled in dogma, but an individual one, which can be found only by relationship with the priest within." [5]

Chiron teaches of the divinity within each and every one of us. *Provers talk of feeling totally connected, of experiencing an inner calm, a trust. Some provers felt connected to the Angelic Realm.* Our western religions have denied us direct contact with the divine, creating another poisonous shadow for the collective unconscious.

5 Anon

Being half God and half horse {unicorn}, he has access to both knowledge of spirit and also wisdom of natural law: a bridge between intellect and intuition. He is known as Chiron the Rainbow Bridge.

Symbolically the rainbow is a bridge between different states of consciousness, life and death, matter and spirit, between one world and another, the meeting of heaven and earth. Created from the union of sunlight and rain, the fire, masculine, spirit, perfectly balanced with the water, feminine, soul. The water splits the light into its separate parts, giving each equal value.

Water, which represents the feeling function, that which values and evaluates; unites with colourless intellectual discrimination and gives it aesthetic substance.

But we have suppressed the feminine and when we search for the feminine myth in our history books and religious texts we find the most powerful women archetypes denigrated to whores and evil witches: Lilith, Mary Magdalene, Morgan le Fey , Jeanne d'Arc and so on. *This issue came up very powerfully during the proving of red, where it is discussed further.*

These myths now neglected and thrown into the darkness of the shadow hold a gift the wisdom of our natural, instinctive existence. This wisdom compliments and animates its opposite of conscious ego.

Everything in light has its opposite dark twin in the shadow. In the Australian Aboriginal tradition the rainbow is not simply an arch in the sky but mirrored in the rainbow snake of the earth. Once again male and female are united in a double rhythm that describes the tension between the masculine and feminine principles in nature. "The rainbow in the sky as visible conscious and available potential, meets the rainbow in the earth, as unknown, unconscious nourisher with limitless potential. For here the personal meets the depths of the collective."[6]

The rainbow snake of the earth and its counterpart in the sky are the same two snakes that balance on our caduceus. After the flood a rainbow is given as a promise from God of completion, wholeness after difficult times.

6 Fruits of the Moon Tree.  Alan Bleakley

However, we are not there yet and the unconscious realm is not an easy place to enter. Accepted laws of reality dissolve as we cross its borders. *Provers found themselves in a different reality, where familiar boundaries such as time and space had no value. In the 'in between time', in an alien dimension, befriending angels, faeries, light beings but also feeling vulnerable to attack from aliens or dark forces. {Like Aids, Arg.nit., Hydr., Nat.c., Nit.ac., Ozone, Phos., Spectrum has an issue with boundaries.} Not surprisingly this brought up many fears including fear of insanity! but in particular both a fear of death coupled with a confrontation with death and an acceptance.* This is appropriate as the doorway into the unconscious is past our fear of personal death, death of the ego, the small self. There can be no transformation without disintegration.

Chiron comes to our aid, a rainbow of hope and a promise of transformation. Having mastered the lessons of Pluto he's happy to guide us into our deepest

wounds, enabling us to transform them and recreate our lives. Chiron brings the potential of healing not just for the individual but also for humanity. As each individual nibbles away at their own shadow, inner mirroring outer, the world will be embued with light and once more we are given the opportunity to realise Heaven on Earth. {Well that's the tale!}

Gill Dransfield

# One Prover's Experiences

A month before we began any of the provings prover No.1 had a series of experiences that I thought were worth recording. She had no knowledge of what we were about to prove and very little knowledge of homeopathy. Here are some excerpts from her diary.

'My first encounter with these souls was during one of my early morning walks with my dog. I cannot remember how it began; one moment I was on a country lane, the next thing I knew I was on a deserted beach waiting and looking towards the sky. Then it started, a shimmering light coming towards me. As it drew nearer I could make out seven tall people who were radiating a beautiful light. There was no fear, just a feeling of peace and love. They were dressed in loose white clothing. One, who appeared to be the elected spokesman, pointed towards the sea and invited me to enter. It was rose pink in colour and as I submerged myself I felt a tremendous feeling of love envelope my body. Emerging from the water I was invited to sit, many beings of light were now seated around me. It was suggested that earth people would be graduating towards a new stage of understanding. As suddenly as they had appeared they left. I was astonished to find that I had been walking for over an hour yet did not remember anything of where I'd walked. These experiences kept recurring'.

'On another morning walk I found myself at the North Pole. My friends who I had first encountered on the beach were there beside me. I was invited to take notice of the landscape; to the right I saw a small igloo. The sky was so, so black and full of stars, the icy snow was gleaming; it was like looking at millions of small lights. As I looked up into the far distance, it began. First a soft light, gradually it began to show itself as colour. I felt the urge to move and dance with this living colour. I was able to pull the colours towards me and then release them at will. I felt a total oneness with all that is, a tremendous power yet a soft gentleness. Just like a mother who lets her young take liberties with her but still has the ability to check'.

'When my dance was at an end I noticed that my garment had taken on all the colours of the rainbow, my face felt radiated. I turned to my companion who invited me into the igloo. I was very surprised to find myself in a very large, white, dome-shaped hall. As I looked around I saw seven archways, vapours of different colours were coming from the archways. I stepped through the first arch into the colour mauve and then through all the other arches through pink, red, yellow, orange, blue and green to observe and learn about the colours…'.

'Finally it was suggested to me that the creative force enters the planet through colour. The North Pole is one of the gateways for this colour. Our earth is a planet of colour and our purpose here is to understand the properties of colour. The colour force comes into our earth and like a mighty network expands itself to incorporate the whole world. It is like looking at a mighty web of rivers. As they flow they energise the mineral kingdom, which in turn gives energy to all of nature, creating a balance in all things. It was suggested to me that we have been interfering with this network via deep mining and nuclear testing, causing breaks and creating disharmony. We are fools if we think we can destroy our planet, only God can take away what he created…'.

'Once again I find myself on a beautiful beach. I'm looking out to sea but it's through a muslin curtain that goes on forever. A gentle breeze lifts the curtain slightly and I stand there looking through the veil. I'm encouraged to slip into the water; it was warm and so blue. As I began to swim a feeling of peace enveloped me. I swam and played in the water and lost myself for an age. I turned and noticed that the light had faded and the moon was full and was casting a silver shimmering path for me to follow. I felt no fear, only peace and the knowledge that I had crossed, in full consciousness, the great divide, the veil that separates life and death…'.

'Walking through my woods one day after all the encounters, I felt a band of little children walking along with me. They were all the same height, and each one radiated a different colour. They had learnt the art of taking on just one particular colour…'.

"...the creative force enters the planet through colour."

Prover 1


Colour is form and form is colour.

Pythagoras

# Science of Spectrum

Deep in the heart of our sun a tiny photon tries to escape, pushing its way through, against the intense pressure of the surrounding atoms undergoing nuclear reaction. Every second approximately six million tonnes of Hydrogen is being 'burnt' at the core of our sun and converted to Helium, our little photon with no mass to speak of, is a product of this intense nuclear fusion. It is estimated that it takes millions of years for the photons created in the dense core to push their way through the mass of the interior to reach the surface of the sun, once there however, travelling at the 'speed of light' they take only 8 minutes to cross the 93,000,000 miles of empty space to reach the surface of our planet.

Equation of the reaction for the conversion of hydrogen to helium plus energy.       $4H \longrightarrow He + Energy$

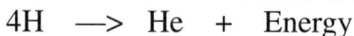

The photon is defined as a Quantum of Light of Electromagnetic Radiation of Energy.       $E = hv$

*[Where h is Plank's Constant and v is the frequency, the rate of repetition or periodicity, measured in Hertz (Cycles per Second)].*

Planks law is the basis of quantum theory, which states that the energy of an electromagnetic waves is confined in indivisible packets or 'quanta', each of which has to be radiated or absorbed as a whole; the magnitude being proportional to the frequency; the higher the frequency, the larger is the Energy and the bigger the quantas of energy.

If $E$ is the value of the quantum expressed in energy units and $v$ is the frequency of the radiation, then $E = hv$. Where $h$ is known as Plank's Constant and has dimensions of Energy times Time. (i.e. Action). The present accepted value is $6.626 \times 10^{-34}$ Joules per second.

The photon has zero rest mass, it weighs nothing when still, if they ever are still, but carries a momentum because of its movement of $hv/c$ where $c$ is the velocity of light.

The introduction of a 'particle' in physics is necessary to explain the photoelectron effect, atomic line spectra, the Compton effect and other properties of electromagnetic radiation.

All electro-magnetic phenomena can have dual properties of both particles and waves.

Electromagnetic waves comprise two interdependent, mutually perpendicular, transverse waves of electric and magnetic fields. The velocity of propagation in free space for all such waves is that of the velocity of light $2.99792458 \times 10^8$ metres per second. The electro-magnetic spectrum ranges from wavelengths of $10^{-15}$ metres to $10^3$ metres, i.e. from gamma rays, through x-rays, ultraviolet, visible light, infrared, microwaves to short, medium and long wave radio-waves.

Electromagnetic waves undergo reflection in mirrors (particles), refraction in prisms, exhibit interference and diffraction effects (waves); they can be polarised as in sunglasses and guided as in fibre optics.

LIGHT is a form of electromagnetic radiation, capable of inducing visual sensation, with wavelengths between 400 to 800 nanometers (0.0000004 to 0.0000008 metres)

Refraction is a phenomenon which occurs when a wave crosses a boundary between two media in which its phase velocity differs, this leads to a change in the direction of the wave front.

"Spectrum" is formed by visible white light from the sun, millions of tiny photons, being passed through a prism and refracted or split into its component bands of light; the colours seen in a rainbow, where sunlight is refracted and internally reflected by raindrops.

From the provings of Hydrogen and Helium by Jeremy Sherr. We see Hydrogen as the soul out of the body, free in the void of space, without boundaries, alone with the stars and God. Helium is the soul coming into the body, incarnation, and awareness of the body, with the desire to find a mission or purpose in life and the need to find ones soul mate.

We see that in nature, in the creation of helium from hydrogen, light is produced. This light might therefore represent the passage of the soul into the body, the journey in and out of life as we change from a spiritual being into a physical existence. It represents the passage into birth or into death, the return of the soul to the void.

This might be an explanation in the accounts of near death experiences, where people talk of a "tunnel of white light", the journey and pathway into and out of life.

Spectrum is the bridge between the spirit and the physical worlds.

David Retford   BSc, Lic. SOH,

PC Hom.

# Methodology of the repertorisation

It seems appropriate to outline the techniques involved in developing the format for a repertorisation. There is necessarily some confusion when collating provers symptoms regarding frequency (how many provers experienced the same thing) and intensity (how often provers experienced the same thing). For the sake of clarity this repertorisation has been based on frequency. The symptoms were collated and then analysed for the purpose of establishing which rubrics would be plain type, italic or bold.

We began considering a 'break point' of 50% for the bold symptoms and 25% for italic. As this did not show much significance we brought the 'break point' down to 40% and 20% respectively. The sample for this proving was quite small—18 provers, so we make no claims to a broad representative sample! However it seems apparent after collating the data that a very clear symptom picture emerges.

Rubric Classification

Plain type = 1-3 provers experienced this symptom.

Italic type = 4-6 provers experienced this symptom.

Bold type = 7+ provers experienced this symptoms.

In order to address the issue of intensity we have designed a single page theme map on page 121. I felt that this would tie together the repertorisation and in the process demonstrate some of the central tenets, which we have found to be highly significant to the Spectrum symptom picture. It has allowed us to present an interpretation of the bigger picture, which is not always so clearly represented in provers notes.

It is hoped that the objective focus on frequency and the more subjective focus on intensity provides a useful overview of the essence of Spectrum.

Dee Lalljee

# Bibliography and Further Reading

Astrology of Fate. ............................................ Liz Greene

Chiron. .......................................................... Barbara Hand Clow

The Dynamics and Methodology
of Homoeopathic Provings. ............................. Jeremy Sherr

In the dark places of Wisdom .......................... Peter Kingsley

Psyche and Substance. .................................... Edward C.Whitmont

An Illustrated Encyclopaedia
of Traditional Symbols. ................................. J.C. Cooper

New Larousse Encyclopaedia of Mythology.

Dictionary of Symbols. ................................... Tom Chetwynd

Fruits of the Moon Tree. ................................. Alan Bleakley

Golden Bough. ............................................... J.G. Frazer

The Greek Myths 1 & 11. ............................... Robert Graves

Colour. .......................................................... Rudolph Steiner

'Synthesis' Edition 7.1 ................................... Dr. Schroyens